Atherosclerosis

THE JONXIS LECTURES

A series of post-graduate medical courses

VOLUME 2

Editorial Board: J.W.F. Beks
Member of the Board of the Foundation for Higher Medical
Education Netherlands Antilles

W. Lammers
Dean of the Medical Faculty, University of Groningen, The
Netherlands

The courses are organized by the 'Foundation for Higher Medical Education
Netherlands Antilles' in cooperation with the Medical Faculty, University of
Groningen, The Netherlands

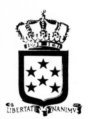 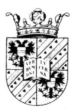

This publication was made possible through the support of the Department for
Netherlands Antilles Affairs, The Hague, The Netherlands

1979
Excerpta Medica, Amsterdam – Oxford

ATHEROSCLEROSIS

Editor:
W.D. Reitsma

Department of Internal Medicine
University Hospital, Groningen, The Netherlands

1979
Excerpta Medica, Amsterdam – Oxford

ISBN Excerpta Medica 90 219 6002 8
ISBN Elsevier North-Holland 0 444 90075 6

Library of Congress Cataloging in Publication Data
Main entry under title:
Atherosclerosis.
  (The Jonxis lectures ; v. 2)
  Includes indexes.
1. Atherosclerosis—Congressess. I. Reitsma, W.D. II. Title. [DNLM: 1. Arteriosclerosis—Congresses. W3 J044 v. 2 / WG550 A8674 1978]
RC692.A727   616.1'36   79-930
ISBN 0-444-90075-6

Publisher:
Excerpta Medica
305 Keizersgracht
1000 BC Amsterdam
P.O. Box 1126

Sole Distributors for the USA and Canada:
Elsevier North-Holland Inc.
52 Vanderbilt Avenue
New York, N.Y. 10017

Printed in the Netherlands by Casparie Alkmaar

Contributors

DR. W.G. VAN AKEN
Departments of Cardiology
and Internal Medicine
University Hospital Wilhelmina Gasthuis
and Department of Blood Coagulation
Central Laboratory of the Netherlands
Red Cross
AMSTERDAM
The Netherlands

PROF. DR. A.C. ARNTZENIUS
Department of Cardiology
Leiden University Hospital
LEIDEN
The Netherlands

PROF. DR. W.H. BIRKENHÄGER
Department of Internal Medicine
Zuiderziekenhuis
ROTTERDAM
The Netherlands

PROF. DR. H. DOORENBOS
Division of Clinical Endocrinology
Department of Internal Medicine
University Hospital
GRONINGEN
The Netherlands

DR. A.J. DUNNING
University Department of Medicine
Binnengasthuis
AMSTERDAM
The Netherlands

DR. A.E. MEINDERS
Department of Internal Medicine
Municipal Hospital
ARNHEM
The Netherlands

PROF. DR. J. NIEVEEN
Department of Cardiology
University Hospital
GRONINGEN
The Netherlands

DR. W.D. REITSMA
Division of Clinical Endocrinology
Department of Internal Medicine
University Hospital
GRONINGEN
The Netherlands

PROF. DR. S. SAILER
Allgemeines Krankenhaus
Universitätsklinik
INNSBRÜCK
Austria

DR. A.E.C. SALEH
Department of Internal Medicine
St. Elisabeth Hospital
WILLEMSTAD – CURAÇAO
Netherlands Antilles

PROF. DR. C.A. WINKEL
Department of Pediatrics
St. Elisabeth Hospital
WILLEMSTAD – CURAÇAO
Netherlands Antilles

The preparation of this book would not have been possible without skilful secretarial help. The congenial assistance of Mrs. G. Dekens-Beuving and Miss J.H. Hettema is acknowledged with appreciation.

Contents

INTRODUCTION

Complications of atherosclerotic vascular disease
like myocardial infarction and cerebrovascular accidents
are nowadays the most frequent causes of death of the modern industrialized world. Decreased physical activity and
abundant food supply are factors, which play an important
role in the increased frequency of atherosclerosis. In the
so-called underdeveloped countries, where people live in
a more natural way, diseases related to atherosclerosis
occur much less frequently. From my own experience, as I
had the opportunity to stay at Curaçao for some time some
years ago, I know that atherosclerotic vascular diseases
are also a major problem in the Caribbean. From this background it is not surprising, that atherosclerosis was
chosen as the subject of a postgraduate course, organized
by the Netherlands-Antillean Foundation for Medical Clinical Education.

The accumulation of cholesteryl esters in the core of
the atheromatous plaque is the most striking abnormality
in human atherosclerosis. Recently progress was made in
the understanding of the significance of abnormalities of
the cholesterol and triglyceride metabolism and of the clotting mechanism in the development of atherosclerosis. To
these fundamental aspects we will give ample attention

1

during this conference. Also the environmental aspects will be discussed.

The primary goal of this conference, however, is a better understanding of the clinical and therapeutical aspects of the diseases, which are related to athero-sclerosis. To this purpose the speakers, representing diverse subspecialties within internal medicine, have been invited. I want to express my hope, that this conference will fulfil the expectations, which the attendants of this meeting have about the presentation of the knowledge on atherosclerosis anno 1978.

W.D. Reitsma.

CHAPTER I

ENVIRONMENTAL FACTORS IN THE DEVELOPMENT

OF ATHEROSCLEROSIS

Arntzenius, A.C.

Introduction

Pathogenesis of atherosclerosis

Risk factors for coronary heart disease

Prevention of coronary heart disease

INTRODUCTION

In most industrialized societies coronary heart disease (CHD) has become very common since the Second World War and it is occurring increasingly early in life.

It is beyond the scope of this presentation to discuss in detail the scientific basis for the belief that coronary atherosclerosis and its clinical consequences, which have now reached epidemic proportions, are due in large part to what people do (the environment) rather than to what they are (the genetic constitution). However, it can scarcely be doubted any longer that susceptibility to CHD is greatly influenced by the daily habits of living.

As a consequence and since mortality from coronary heart disease has not substantially been influenced by the introduction of coronary care units, surgical intervention and first aid ambulances, the only approach that is likely to have a real impact on the disease will be prevention.

Prevention of coronary heart disease requires that the disease is predicted from its forerunners: the risk factors. If we wait for early symptoms we are likely to be too late, since the earliest clinical manifestation of the disease may at the same time be its last one, namely death.

Coronary heart disease

In The Netherlands in 1974, 45.7 % of all deaths were due to cardiovascular disease and 45 % of these stem from coronary heart disease. Coronary heart disease, once it has become clinically manifest, impairs or threatens life. The life expectation of those fortunate enough to survive a myocardial infarction or of those with angina pectoris is shortened five times. At least a quarter of the patients with a heart attack die before reaching the hospital and are thus unable to benefit from treatment in a coronary care unit.

Quite clearly then, CHD has a high degree of prevalence in The Netherlands, and it is also of serious consequences to the individual.

Coronary heart disease in Europe

Cardiovascular diseases constitute the leading cause of death in Europe as in most so-called developed, i.e., industrialized parts of the world. The most common cardiovascular diseases are coronary heart disease and other clinical consequences of atherosclerosis. They account for between 30 and 40 per cent of all deaths, more than any other single cause. Amongst men, no less than a third or more of coronary heart disease deaths occur prior to age 65. Coronary heart disease is less frequent amongst women and their life expectancy is correspondingly greater, but this trend may be changing.

Coronary heart disease in The United States

In The United States the number of deaths from atherosclerosis steadily increased during the World War II and in the years thereafter. The age-adjudged death rate from coronary heart disease however, has peaked in 1963 and has declined since (Walker[1], 1974).

In 1977 the figures of the National Center for Health Statistics of the United States showed that in all age groups from 35-74 years, between 1963 and 1975 there was a percentage decline in coronary mortality of around 18 %.

5

PATHOGENESIS OF ATHEROSCLEROSIS

Two very important theories have since long prevailed on this subject: the lipid infiltration and elimination theory and secondly the theory on damage of the arterial wall with consequently clotting mechanisms to set in.

The lipid theory, originated by Virchow[2] in 1862, will have it that fatty substances from the blood, filtrate into the arterial wall. This theory quite in a natural way "explains" the high degree of atherosclerosis with fatty infiltrations in the arterial wall in the presence of hyperlipidemia and elevated bloodpressure (which pushes the lipids to the other side of the intimal layer).

Also, many investigations since Virchow's days have analyzed the relationship between serum cholesterol and arterial atherosclerosis.

Gofman[3] (1954) with the use of the ultracentrifuge distinguished different classes of lipoproteins. Elevated LDL (Low Density Lipoproteins) have proven to be the most important contributors to early coronary sclerotic lesions (Frederickson type II). Cholesterol elevations resulting from too much VLDL (Very Low Density Lipoproteins) probably contribute to peripheral arteriosclerotic narrowing.

Recently, the HDL (High Density Lipoproteins) fraction has been shown by Miller and Miller[4] to be inversely related to atherosclerosis: the higher the HDL-cholesterol content of the blood the less chance to develop clinical manifestations of the disease.

The theory that atherosclerosis finds its origin particularly due to damage of the arterial wall stems from Rokitansky[5] (1852) and Duguid[6] (1946).

Clotting of platelets at the site of injury is supposed to play an important role and indeed patients with ischemic disease are found to have platelets that aggregate more easily than those in normal individuals. Each little place of damage can thus cause platelet adhesion and later bleeding in the wall.

This theory can easily "explain" why arterial sclerotic lesions often are found at places where the arteries divide and where they are apt to move about a great deal.

Also, the fact that smokers tend to develop arteriosclerotic diseases so often can be thought to be due to small lesions as both carbonoxyde and nicotine have been shown to damage the arterial wall with formation of local edema.

Once platelets adhere the local damaged intimal wall and when bleedings occur in the interna, it is quite understandable that thrombus forming will eventually block the arterial lumen at those sites. Those who adhere to the above theory will try and influence the process by providing for anticoagulant treatment and by prescribing drugs such as aspirin which supposedly can reduce platelet cohesion and adherence.

RISK FACTORS FOR CORONARY HEART DISEASE

What is a risk factor?

The risk factor was developed when it became apparent that, on the basis of such variables as serum cholesterol, bloodpressure, and smoking, a heart attack could be predicted with a known degree of probability in clinically well people. A "risk factor" is a factor associated with the development of the disease. The risk factor concept does not necessarily imply that elimination of the risk factor will lower the risk of disease. However, recommendations on preventing coronary heart disease are based on the assumption that there is cause-and-effect relationship between risk factor and the disease.

Serum cholesterol

All prospective surveys on risk factors for CHD have confirmed the findings of the Framingham study that risk for future clinical manifestations of coronary sclerosis rises continuously with increasing serum cholesterol level.
Serum cholesterol levels depend largely on the saturated fat and on the cholesterol content of the diet. Serum cholesterol levels can be controlled by means of modified-fat diets.

Serum HDL-cholesterol

Recently it has been shown that a low HDL cholesterol level carries with it an increased risk for CHD (T. Gordon[7], 1977 and M.E. Miller[8], 1977).
HDL-cholesterol has therefore been called a negative risk factor: the higher its serum level the less chance for future CHD. Women have higher mean levels than men.
As regards its mechanism Miller and Miller[4] have proposed that a reduction of plasma HDL concentration may accelerate the development of atherosclerosis by impairing the clearance of cholesterol from the arterial wall.

Serum triglycerides

Serum triglycerides when elevated probably carry a small risk for atherosclerosis which is independent of serum cholesterol. It seems to be related to future peripheral atherosclerotic lesions. Serum triglycerides when elevated usually are accompanied by (if only moderate) elevation of serum cholesterol.

Blood Pressure

Elevated bloodpressure constitutes a major risk for CHD. It rises continuously with increasing pressure. Systolic pressure is as predictive as the diastolic one.

A single reading in itself is insufficient basis on which to establish the diagnosis of hypertension. Active intervention requires at least two measurements of two separate days.

Cigarette smoking

Smoking of cigarettes carries a high risk which is independent of cholesterol and blood pressure level. On an average the risk for a smoker is double that for non-smoker.

Smokers generally die 7 years earlier than non-smokers. In persons who have stopped smoking the risk becomes reduced to that of non-smokers within a few years. Cigarette smokers who switch to pipes and cigars frequently continue to inhale the smoke and probably gain little from the change.

Diabetes and glucose intolerance

There is no doubt that diabetic men and women have an excessive risk developing coronary heart disease.

Glucose intolerance probably also constitutes a slight increased coronary risk. Clinically manifest or

latent diabetes should be treated preferably by diet
alone if possible.

Obesity

Obesity on the whole indicates an increase in risk
for CHD. Much of the risk associated with obesity however,
is due to the fact that obese persons often have hypertension, hyperlipidemia or glucose intolerance.

Stress

Some investigations indicate that subjects characterized by a strong sense of urgency speed of work and high
job involvement ("type A") are more prone to coronary
heart disease than the reverse type ("type B"). Also,
stress, no matter how it is defined, may be an important
risk factor for some persons.
Stress however remains difficult to detect and to
modify. Control of other risk factors in persons under
stress will be very important.

Oral contraceptives

Recently two groups[9)10)] of workers found in prospective studies that oral contraceptive users have shown
an increased mortality from diseases of the circulatory
system.
The "pill" has been shown to raise the levels of
serum triglycerides, cholesterol, the bloodpressure. It
seems wise therefore if a woman is hypertensive, hyperlipidemic or hyperglycemic not to prescribe oral contraceptives.

Physical inactivity

Prevalence and incidence of CHD are generally lower among people engaged in regular physical activity than among those physically inactive. Physical activity may lower bloodpressure but it has no substantial effect on serum cholesterol.

PREVENTION OF CORONARY HEART DISEASE (CHD)

General remarks

One of the most important statements as regards coronary heart disease ever made is William Kannel's[11] one in 1976 which reads: "Most cases of angina pectoris or myocardial infarctions represent medical failures; the conditions should have been detected years earlier for preventive management".

Indeed, atherosclerosis begins slowly at an early age and some 20 or 30 years later clinical manifestations of a very serious nature develop, either slowly or abruptly.

During those 20 or 30 years not only do we have time to detect the forerunners of atherosclerosis: its risk factors, but also, there is ample time to lower the risk with harmless non-drug intervention techniques, quite acceptable to the general public.

Prevention

The most striking example of succesful prevention has been given by the general population of the United States. Around the early 1950's, it was suggested that the public should curtail its intake of butterfat and high cholesterol foods in order to reduce the number of coronary deaths. In 1964 the surgeon general issued a warning concerning the health hazards of cigarette smoking.

From 1963 to 1975 there has been a decline in the pro-capita consumption in the US of tobacco (22 %), animal fats and oils (56 %), butter (32 %), fluid milk and cream (19 %) and eggs (12 %) with an associated increase in consumption of vegetable fats and oils (44 %). There is no doubt that these changed smoking and eating habits were the principle basis for the decline in age specific coronary mortality as reported by Walker[1], which amount to around 18 % for age groups 35-74 years in the period 1963-1975. Coronary mortality at present drops in the USA with a steady 2 % per year.

The second very important quotation I would like to use is one of Weldon Walker[12] when in 1976 he states: "The success during the past 10 years suggests that much more can be accomplished with present knowledge and we must use this knowledge more effectively". So as to gather more knowledge both as regards the mechanisms of preventive measures and as regards their acceptability many studies have been undertaken of which I would like to review a few.

As regards secundary prevention, Paul Leren's Oslo[13] study should be mentioned here.

It dealt with 412 men (30-64 years) 1-2 years after established myocardial infarction. Randomization provided for a dietary versus a non-treated group.

Diet consisted of little saturated fat, cholesterol (264 mg/day) and a P/S ratio of 2.4, total fat: 37 cal %. After 5 years, incidence in fatal as well as in non-fatal reinfarction was significantly lower in the treated group.

12

The serum cholesterol dropped in the treated group with 17.6 % (controls: 3.7 %).

As regards primary prevention two major trials are on their way in the US.

Lipid clinics type II coronary primary prevention trial [14] is sponsored by the National Heart and Lung Institute.

Its object is to lower serum cholesterol in type II patients with diet and cholestyramine (24 g/day).

500,000 individuals were screened to find the necessary 3,600 patients with serum cholesterol: > 265 mg %, LDL cholesterol: > 190 mg % and triglycerides: > 300 mg %. Hypertensive and obese patients were excluded. There will be a randomized treatment group and all coronary events will be registered. Total costs: $ 58 x 10^6.

The MRFIT (Multiple Risk Factor Intervention Trial) [15] has also recently started under supervision of the National Heart and Lung Institute. It is a six year primary prevention study involving approximately 12,000 participants aged 35-57 years. The participants are in the upper 15 % of the population distribution for risk for CHD as determined by cholesterol levels, bloodpressure and degree of cigarette smoking by the Framingham study predictions of risk. Half of the group is to be followed-up by their usual source of medical care and half will receive a specific intervention programme. Total costs around $ 112 x 10^6.

The CB Heart Project (Netherlands) [16] [17] [18]
In The Netherlands a community project on the acceptability and efficacy of risk factor lowering techniques was instituted in 1973, first in three and later in six consultation bureaus for tuberculosis. In this project in

the period March '73 to September '74 8,000 individuals
were enrolled via a screening examination. Of those enrolled, 1,975 persons identified with high risk for developing coronary heart disease (CHD) could be followed-up
during one year of intervention and periodic re-examination.
Attendance rate was 80 % and coverage rate of high risk
persons to intervention programma was 89 %. Seven public
health nurses trained for the purpose, instructed each
high risk person on the average 6 times, either in the
consultation bureau or at home. Intervention consisted of
hygienic and dietary measures. Results on "elevated" risks
only, were as follows:

	No	Unit	at entry	after 1 year	"pure" change[*]
Cholesterol	510	mmol/l	8.0	7.0	− 8 %
Syst. B.P.	156	mm Hg	170	145	− 9 %
Diast. B.P.	50	mm Hg	110	92	− 12 %
Cig. smoking	386	cig/day	29	18	− 37 %

[*] adjusted for "regression to the mean"

Of the high risk group at final examination 54 % had
either moved to borderline risk (35 %) or could be classified as low risks (19 %), which can be considered as
satisfactory.

We would like to conclude from the preventive projects
and trials that no longer is it justified to withhold preventive instructions from those who are at the greatest
risk: those with two or more elevated risk factors. Also,
the general public in Europe and everywhere should be
given the same information as regards food substances and
warnings concerning health hazards of smoking as has been
given to the US public.

REFERENCES

1. Walker, W.J. Coronary mortality: What is going on?
    JAMA, 227, 1045-1046, 1974.
2. Virchow, R. Gesammelte Abhandlungen zur Wissenschaft-
    lichen Medizin. Berlin Max Hirsch, 1862.
3. Gofman, J.W., Delalla, O., Glazier, F., Freeman, N.K.,
    Lindgren, F.T., Nichols, A.V., Strisower, B., Tamplin,
    A.R. The serum lipoprotein transport system in health
    metabolic disorders, atherosclerosis and coronary
    heart disease. Plasma, 2, 413-484, 1954.
4. Miller, G.J., Miller, N.E. Plasma-high-density lipo-
    protein concentration and development of ischaemic
    heart disease. Lancet, 1, 16-19, 1975.
5. Rokitansky, C. A manual of pathological anatomy.
    (Trans. by George E. Day, London Sydenham Society),
    Vol. 4, 261-272, 1852.
6. Duguid, J.B. Thrombosis as a factor in the pathogenesis
    of coronary atherosclerosis. J. Path. Bact., 58, 207-
    212, 1946.
7. Gordon, T. High density lipoprotein as a protective
    factor against coronary heart disease. The Framingham
    Study. The American Journal of Medicine, 62, 707-714,
    1977.
8. Miller, N.E., Thelle, D.S., Førde, O.H., Mjøs, O.D.
    The Tromsø Heart-Study. The Lancet, 965-967, 1977.
9. Royal College of General Practitioners: Oral Contra-
    ception Study. Mortality among oral-contraceptive users.
    The Lancet, 727-731, 8 oct. 1977.
10. Vessey, M.P., McPherson, K., Johnson, B. Mortality
    among women participating in the Oxford family planning
    association contraceptive study. The Lancet, 731-733,
    8 oct. 1977.

11. Kannel, W.B. Some lessons in cardiovascular epidemiology from Framingham. The American Journal of Cardiology, *37*, 269-282, 1976.

12. Walker, W.J. Success story: The programme against major cardiovascular risk factors. Geriatrics, *31*, 97-104, 1976.

13. Leren, P. The effect of plasma cholesterol lowering diet in male survivors of myocardial infarction - a controlled clinical trial. Acta Med. Scan. Supplement 466, 1966.

14. Rifkind, B.M. Lipid clinics type II coronary primary prevention trial (Abstract W-96). The IVth International Symposium on Atherosclerosis, Tokyo, Japan, August 24-28, 1976.

15. MRFIT. The multiple risk factor intervention trial. A national study of primary prevention of coronary heart disease. JAMA, *235*, 825-827, 1976.

16. Sluyter, D.P., Arntzenius, A.C., Meyer, J., Styblo, K. CB heart project in The Netherlands. Population under study and methods of intervention. Hartbulletin, *8*, 42-46, 1977.

17. Styblo, K., Arntzenius, A.C., Van Geuns, H.A., De Haas, J.H., Mellema, T.L., Meyer, J., Sluyter, D.P. CB Heart project in The Netherlands. Reduction of coronary risk factors in a general population. Circulation abstracts, 53 and 54, suppl. II, II-226, 1976.

18) Arntzenius, A.C., Styblo, K., Meyer, J., Sluyter, D.P. Intervention results in high risk individuals of the CB heart project in The Netherlands. State of prevention and therapy in human arteriosclerosis and in animal models. Abhandlungen der Rheinisch-Westfälischen Akademie der Wissenschaften. Band 63, 1978, Westdeutscher Verlag GmbH, Opladen.

CHAPTER II

BLOOD COAGULATION, THROMBOSIS AND ATHEROSCLEROSIS

Van Aken, W.G.

INTRODUCTION

Atherosclerotic lesions are characterized by intimal
proliferation of smooth muscle cells, accumulation of connective tissue material and deposition of intra- and
extracellular lipid. Many factors are involved in this
process, but only the contribution of blood coagulation and
in particular platelets, is discussed here.

Historically, it is of interest that a relationship
between blood coagulation and atherosclerosis was already
proposed by Rokitansky in 1852. He believed that the fundamental change in atherosclerosis was the deposition of
an endogenous product derived from the blood - and for the
most part from fibrin - in the arterial wall which later
underwent metamorphosis into a pulpy mass. This theory,
called encrustation or thrombogenic theory, was revived
almost a century later by Duguid (1946) who concluded that
many of the lesions classified as atherosclerotic were in
fact arterial thrombi which had been converted to fibrous
thickenings.

During the last few years, it has become apparent
that indeed platelets and blood coagulation may contribute to the development of occlusive arterial disease in
several ways. Thrombi, either occlusive or mural, and pla-

telet emboli may form in association with advanced atherosclerosis. Furthermore, endothelial injury and the response of smooth muscle cells to vessel damage, appear to
be early events in the development of atherosclerosis and
both seem to be mediated through platelets. These aspects
will be elaborated in the following discussion but before
this, it seems advisable to summarize what is currently
known concerning the formation of arterial thrombosis.
Several detailed reviews on this subject have been published (Weiss, 1975; Mustard and Packham, 1975; Mustard,
1976; Ross and Glomset, 1976; Harker, 1976).

Thrombus formation

The most important factors involved in thrombus formation appear to be vessel wall injury, platelet adhesion
and aggregation, activation of blood clotting factors
causing fibrin formation, changes in blood flow and possibly also leukocyte reactions. Arterial and venous thrombi differ from one another in their relative amounts of
platelets, leukocytes, erythrocytes and fibrin. Whereas
arterial thrombi are mainly composed of platelets, thrombi
on the venous side form in slowly flowing blood and consist mainly of fibrin and red cells (Table I). In this
review, only the formation of arterial thrombosis will be
discussed.

The initial event in thrombus formation is the adherence of platelets to the subendothelium of the vessel wall
after endothelial damage has occurred. Platelet adhesion
to subendothelial collagen initiates a secretory process,
the so-called release reaction, during which subcellular
granules from platelets escape in the surrounding plasma
or tissues. Among the substances released is adenosine di-

18

TABLE 1 - Comparison between arterial and venous thrombus formation

Contributing factor	Venous thrombosis	Arterial thrombosis
Blood flow (stasis)	++	−
Vessel wall injury	±	++
Platelets	+	++
Blood clotting (fibrin)	++	+
Leukocytes	+	+
Fibrinolysis	++	±

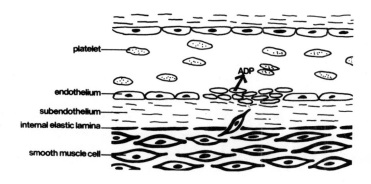

Fig. 1. Platelet adhesion and release reaction

phosphate (ADP) which can directly aggregate platelets. Platelet aggregation causes the mural platelet accretion to become larger and extend into the vessel lumen. The platelet thrombus, which is thus formed, is still unstable and may give rise to multiple emboli or continue to build up until it has effects on the local blood flow. When the

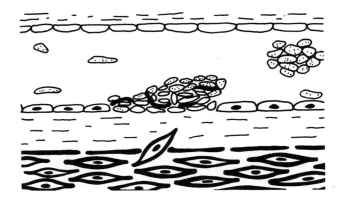

Fig. 2. Platelet, aggregation and embolization

latter occurs and thrombin is formed, platelets at the periphery of the mass undergo morphological changes, termed viscous metamorphosis. Furthermore, leukocytes adhere to platelet aggregates and fibrin can be detected. Thereby, the thrombus is stabilized, permitting further growth through deposition of more platelets and fibrin. When the vessel lumen becomes occluded, the blood distally and proximally to the occlusion clots, giving this component the appearance of a blood clot. From experimental studies, it appears that many arterial thrombi will not reach this stage but remain mural. Approximately one week after endothelial injury has occurred, the vessel is relined with cells similar to endothelial cells. Few remnants of the platelet deposit can be identified, but the intima is thickened by migration of smooth muscle cells from the media through lacunae in the internal elastic lamina to the subendothelium. This process is still reversible, but when the new endothelium is removed by a second injury, an augmented response is induced which is characterized by the formation of an increased number of platelet thrombi, accumulation of fibrin and migration and proliferation of smooth muscle cells (Stemerman, 1974). The resulting lesion is very similar to the early atherosclerotic lesion, known as the fibro-muscular plaque.

Since this latter evidence indicates that repeated injury to the endothelium and the subsequent interaction between blood components and vascular tissues, may be important in the development of atherosclerotic lesions, these reactions will be discussed more in detail in the following paragraphs.

Vessel wall injury

Data obtained from experimental studies and from post-mortem human material indicate that sites of early vessel wall changes associated with atherosclerosis represent areas of vessel injury. Disruption of the endothelial barrier can be observed by study of the uptake of dyes, such as Evans blue. The intensity of the stain is considered to be proportional to endothelial permeability, the degree of endothelial injury or both (Jorgensen et al., 1972). The sites that show the greatest accumulation of the stain, such as around vessel branches, are also the sites at which atherosclerosis tends to develop. In addition, these areas show increased endothelial cell turnover as indicated by the increased incorporation of radioactive thymidine.

There are many agents and conditions that may induce endothelial injury. These include hemodynamic forces, bacteria, viruses, endotoxin, antigen-antibody complexes, epinephrine, cholesterol, homocystine, carbon monoxide and anoxia. Blood platelets may contribute to endothelial injury in areas of disturbed flow where they form aggregates and release platelet factors that increase vessel permeability.

Platelet reactions to vascular injury

Under normal conditions, platelets ignore the endothelium, but once this is damaged platelet adhesion occurs. The mechanisms involved in platelet adhesion to subendothelial structures are still poorly understood, but platelet membrane sulfhydryl groups and glycosyl transferase present in the platelet membrane appear important (Jamieson et al., 1971).

Upon adherence to subendothelial collagen, the platelets undergo a series of reactions (Fig. 3).

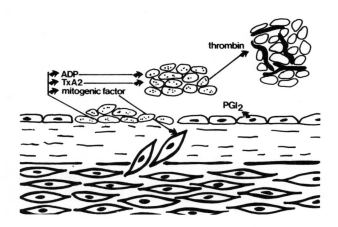

Fig. 3. Thrombus-formation

1. They change from disks to swollen spheres, aggregate with adjacent platelets and progress to the release reaction. During this reaction, the contents of platelet granules, including ADP, ATP, serotonin, epinephrine, calcium, fibrinogen, lysosomal enzymes and a mitogenic factor for smooth muscle cells, escape. ADP is of special importance since it was shown that the addition of this nucleotide to blood results in platelet aggregation. Thus, the primary induced platelet aggregation by collagen is followed by secondary platelet aggregation due to the release of endogenous ADP.

2. When platelets are stimulated by collagen, arachidonic acid, probably made available by hydrolysis of platelet membrane phospholipid, is converted by a cyclo-oxygenase to prostaglandin endoperoxides (PGG_2 and PGH_2) and thromboxane A_2 (see Scheme 1) (Smith et al., 1973; Samuelsson et al., 1976). These unstable intermediates of the prostaglandin pathway are themselves aggregating and release inducing agents that may augment the collagen-induced aggregation.

3. Although the primary adhesion and aggregation of platelets are independent of blood coagulation, there is no doubt that thrombin formation influences the growth and stability of the platelet thrombus. Thrombin formation is probably mediated by humoral coagulation factors and a number of coagulant activities that are associated with platelets. Platelet factor 3, the well-known capacity of platelets to catalyze the reactions of clotting factors X_a and V to activate prothrombin to thrombin, becomes available during platelet aggregation. In addition, platelets were shown to contain intrinsic factor X_a-forming activity (by which factors XI_a, VIII and IX are catalyzed to

activate factor X) and a contact product forming activity, both of which may initiate intrinsic blood coagulation after platelets have responded to ADP (Walsh, 1973). The generation of such products may lead to thrombin formation and ultimately to fibrin formation. In this way, the platelet aggregate serves as a site for the local generation of thrombin, which may cause further platelet aggregation

S C H E M E 1

PROSTAGLANDIN METABOLISM IN PLATELETS

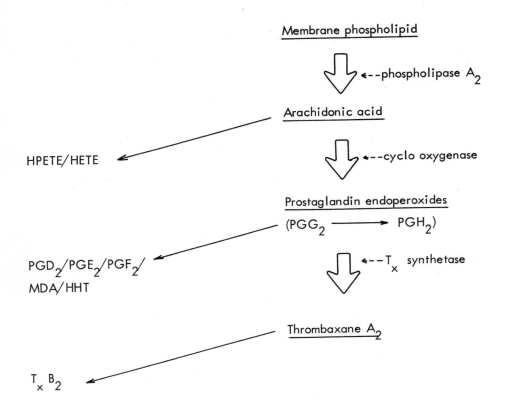

and release of platelet constituents. Thrombin-induced platelet aggregation involves the release of ADP, activation of the arachidonate pathway and one or more additional mechanisms (Kinlough-Rathbone et al., 1977); the latter, as yet not defined, mechanisms are not inhibited by most platelet function inhibiting drugs. Thrombin also activates clotting factors and converts fibrinogen into fibrin which stabilizes the platelet mass, since platelets adhere to polymerizing fibrin (Niewiarowski et al., 1972).

Vessel wall response to thrombosis

When the endothelium is injured, plasma constituents, blood cells and products derived from blood cells can penetrate into the subendothelial spaces. Platelets release materials that increase endothelial permeability (Moncada et al., 1973; Kuehl et al., 1977) and cause vascular contraction (Ellis et al., 1976). Furthermore, collagenase and elastase, which alter the connective tissue in the vessel wall, become available at the platelet surface during the release reaction (Legrand et al., 1973; Chesney et al., 1974).

Probably most important for the development of atherosclerosis is the observation that platelets form or release a factor which is mitogenic for smooth muscle cells (Ross and Glomset, 1973). This mitogenic factor is likely to be involved in the migration and subsequent proliferation of smooth muscle cells from the media which occurs 5 to 7 days after intimal injury. The proliferating cells, surrounded by newly formed collagen and elastic fibers, cause intimal thickening. The importance of the platelet mitogenic factor was first shown in arterial smooth muscle cell cultures (Ross et al., 1974) and thereafter confirmed

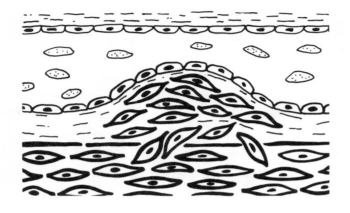

Fig. 4. Smooth muscle cell proliferation

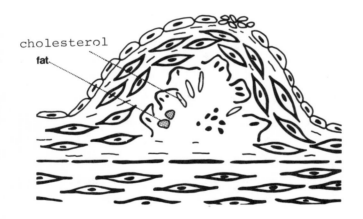

cholesterol

fat

Fig. 5. Advanced atherosclerotic plaque

in thrombocytopenic animals in which smooth muscle proliferation after endothelial injury was dramatically inhibited (Friedman et al., 1977). Although the platelet factor appears to be required to trigger cell proliferation, serum low-density lipoproteins and insulin have a supportive role (Ross and Glomset, 1976).

These and other findings have led Ross and Glomset to modify the so-called 'response to injury' hypothesis, originally proposed by Virchow, in order to clarify the pathogenesis of atherosclerosis.

This hypothesis (Ross and Glomset, 1976) proposes that focal injury to the endothelium both alters endothelial permeability and leads to desquamation of endothetial cells at sites of injury. The exposure of subendothelial connective tissue will cause platelets to adhere and aggregate, a process that is followed by release of platelet granules. The physiological response of platelet release results in the entrance of platelet factors into the arterial wall together with plasma constituents, such as lipoproteins, causing migration and proliferation of smooth muscle cells at the sites of injury. This smooth muscle cell proliferation would be accompanied by the synthesis and secretion of connective tissue proteins and the intra- and extracellular deposition of lipids. Furthermore, the hypothesis proposes that restoration of the endothelial barrier would lead to regression of the lesions whereas repeated endothelial injury would enhance smooth muscle proliferation and lipid accumulation. Consequently, the balance between cell proliferation and cell destruction, which determines whether the lesion enlarges or shows regression, would be regulated by the integrity of the overlying endothelium.

This hypothesis has been tested in 2 experimental animal (baboon) models. In one of these, it was found that chronic hyperlipidemia results not only in the de - position of lipids in the atheromatous lesions, but that it may produce the primary endothelial injury that initiates the process of atherosclerosis as well (Ross and Harker, 1976). Furthermore, platelet survival was significantly shortened in hyperlipidemic animals, which correlated directly with the amount of endothelium removed. A decrease in platelet survival is of particular interest in view of earlier observations by Harker et al. (1976) that baboons made homocystinemic had decreased platelet survival and also developed lesions of atherosclerosis identical to fibrous plaques. When chronically homocystinemic baboons were treated with dipyridamole, a platelet-function inhibiting drug, platelet survival became normal and intimal proliferation lesions showed a striking reduction, although the focal desquamation of the endothelium persisted. Thus, after different forms of injury, the role of platelets appears to be critical in inducing the smooth muscle cell proliferation response. The response-to-injury hypothesis offers the possibility to investigate the mechanisms by which other risk factors (hypertension, smoking, diabetes) affect the development of vascular disease. Furthermore, it will be of interest to study the mechanisms whereby vascular lesions possibly regress either 'spontaneously' or by drug treatment.

Thromboembolic complications of atherosclerosis

In areas of disturbed bloow flow, embolization of thrombotic material is likely to occur as long as the initial platelet thrombus, which is formed after endothelial

injury, is not stabilized. Experimentally, it has been
shown that transient platelet aggregates in the microcirculation of the myocardium can cause cardiac arrythmia and
sudden death (Jorgensen et al., 1967). Similarly, chronic
nephrosclerosis and hypertension may develop when platelet
emboli are formed in the aorta above the renal arteries
(Moore, 1973). Intravascular platelet aggregates were also
observed after infusion of norepinephrine (Haft et al.,
1972) and in the microcirculation distally to electrically
induced thrombosis of the coronary arteries of dogs
(Moschos et al., 1972). These experimental data demonstrate
that not only occlusive arterial disease may cause organ
damage but that, prior to vascular occlusion, thromboembolic complications of vascular injury (e.g. by atherosclerosis) may give rise to ischemia. This is potentially
relevant to clinical situations, such as impending myocardial infarction, transient cerebral ischemic attacks
and amourosis fugax, where atherosclerosis may be complicated by the formation of platelet emboli (Fig. 6).

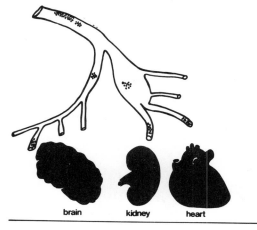

brain   kidney   heart

Fig. 6. Thromboembolic complications of atherosclerosis

The information on the relation between thrombosis and atherosclerosis presented thus far is mainly derived from experimental in vitro and in vivo studies. Already for a number of years, a relationship has been sought between alterations in platelet function and blood clotting factors on one side and a tendency to develop thrombosis on the other. The observations that factors, such as smoking, certain blood groups and oral contraceptives, predispose to various kinds of thrombosis, notably in young people, support the hypothesis that such blood abnormalities may exist. Moreover, there are reports of a familial tendency to develop venous thrombosis and pulmonary embolism caused by antithrombin III deficiency (Egeberg, 1965; van der Meer et al., 1973; Marciniak et al., 1974). A striking tendency for arterial thrombosis is, however, not observed in this condition. Patients with thrombocytosis (Zucker and Mielke, 1972), thrombocythemia (Preston et al., 1974) and spontaneous platelet aggregation (Vreeken and van Aken, 1971) are known to develop venous as well as arterial thrombosis. Homocystinemia, an inborn error of metabolism due to a deficiency of the enzyme cystathione synthase, is manifested clinically by a high frequency of arterial thrombo-embolism and atherosclerosis in combination with congenital deformities (Harker et al., 1974). In these patients platelet turnover was found to be increased.

These disturbances are, however, not frequent. The application of several in vitro platelet function tests in the evaluation of arterial thrombotic disease has up till now not been of diagnostic or predictive value. It should appear, however, that measurement of in vivo platelet survival shows more promise. Platelet survival appears to be shortened in patients with arterial thrombosis, homocystinemia and in patients with valvular heart disease, who have a history of thromboembolic complications (Harker and Slichter, 1972; Weily et al., 1974; Steele et al., 1974; Harker et al., 1974). Recently, circulating platelet aggregates have been demonstrated in patients with transient cerebral ischemic attacks (Wu and Hoak, 1975).

Finally, investigations of patients with congenital hemorrhagic diathesis, either by clotting factor deficiencies or platelet abnormalities, could also help to shed light on the pathogenesis of thrombosis and athero-sclerosis. No data are available on the presence and extent of atherosclerosis in patients with congenital platelet disorders, such as thrombasthenia in which platelets fail to aggregate upon addition of ADP. Atherosclerosis has been described to occur in patients with hemophilia A and B (Stewart and Acheson, 1957; Borchgrevink, 1959; Brody and Beizer, 1965) and also in patients with von Willebrand's disease (Silwer et al., 1966), a genetic disorder characterized by prolongation of the bleeding time, factor VIII deficiency and disturbed platelet function. The latter finding, however, contrasts with the reduced frequency of atherosclerosis which is observed in adult pigs with von Willebrand's disease (Fuster et al., 1978).

These data suggest that certain congenital blood clotting disturbances, which are associated with hemorrhagic diathesis, do not necessarily protect against the development of atherosclerosis. Furthermore, arterial thrombosis is not a predominant feature in patients with an abnormal blood clotting tendency (e.g. antithrombin III deficiency) which causes recurrent venous thrombosis.

It appears, however, that increased arterial thrombosis and atherosclerosis occur when platelet function is abnormal. Thus, one may speculate that the contribution of platelet reactions to atherosclerosis is more important than the role of fibrin formation.

CONCLUSION

Until recently, thrombus formation was frequently considered to be synonymous with blood clotting. Though this may be correct in venous thrombosis, in arterial thrombosis it is a relatively late sequela rather than a primary event. By adhesion to the injured vessel wall and subsequent aggregation, platelets may initiate and sustain arterial thrombosis. In addition, platelets may increase vessel wall permeability and release a mitogenic factor which induces the proliferation of smooth muscle cells which have emigrated from the media to the intima. Since smooth muscle cell proliferation appears to be a prominent feature of atherosclerosis, pharmacologically-induced alteration of platelet function may offer promising new leads in the prevention and therapy of arterial occlusive disease.

REFERENCES

1. Borgrevink, C.F. Myocardial infarction in a haemophilic. Lancet, 1, 1229, 1959.
2. Brody, J.S., Beizer, L.M. Christmas disease and myocardial infarction. Arch. Intern. Med., 115, 552, 1965.
3. Chesney, C.M., Harper, E., Colman, R.W. Human platelet collagenase. J. Clin. Invest., 53, 1647, 1974.

4. Duguid, J.B. Thrombosis as a factor in the pathogenesis of coronary thrombosis. J. Path. Bact., 58, 207, 1946.

5. Egeberg, O. Inherited antithrombin deficiency causing thrombophilia. Thromb. Diath. Hemorrh., 13, 516, 1965.

6. Ellis, E.F., Oelz, O., Roberts, L.J., Payne, N.A., Sweetman, B.J., Nies, A.S., Oates, J.A. Coronary arterial smooth muscle contraction by a substance released from platelets. Science, 193, 1135, 1976.

7. Friedman, R.J., Stemerman, M.B., Wenz, B., Moore, S., Gauldie, J., Gent, M., Tiell, M.L., Spaet, Th.H. The effect of thrombocytopenia on experimental lesion formation in rabbits. J. Clin. Invest., 60, 1191, 1977.

8. Fuster, V., Bowie, E.J., Lewis, J.C., Fass, D.N., Owen, C.A., Brown, A.L. Resistance to arteriosclerosis in pigs with von Willebrand's disease. J. Clin. Invest., 61, 722, 1978.

9. Haft, J.I., Kranz, P.D., Albert, F.J., Fani, K. Intravascular platelet aggregation in the heart induced by norepinephrine. Circulation, 46, 698, 1972.

10. Harker, L.A., Ross, R., Slichter, S., Scott, C. Homocystine-induced atherosclerosis: The role of endothelial cell injury and platelet response in its genesis. J. Clin. Invest., 58, 731, 1976.

11. Harker, L.A., Slichter, S.J. Platelet and fibrinogen consumption in man. New Engl. J. Med., 287, 999, 1972.

12. Harker, L.A., Slichter, S.J., Scott, C.R., Ross, R. Homocystinemia: Vascular injury and arterial thrombosis. New Engl. J. Med., 291, 537, 1974.

13. Jamieson, G.A., Urban, C.L., Barber, A.J. Enzymatic basis for platelet-collagen adhesion as the primary step in hemostasis. Nature New Biol., 234, 5, 1971.

14. Jorgensen, L., Packham, M.A., Rowsell, H.C., Mustard, J.F. Deposition of formed elements of blood on the intima and signs of intimal injury in the aorta of rabbit, pig and man. Lab. Invest., _27_, 341, 1972.

15. Jorgensen, L., Rowsell, H.C., Hovig, T., Glynn, M.F., Mustard, J.F. Adenosine diphosphate-induced platelet aggregation and myocardial infarction in swine. Lab. Invest., _17_, 616, 1967.

16. Kuehl, F.A., Humes, J.L., Egan, R.W., Ham, E.A., Beveridge, G.C., van Armon, C.G. Role of prostaglandin endoperoxide PGG_2 in inflammatory processes. Nature, _265_, 170, 1977.

17. Legrand, Y., Caen, J.P., Booyse, F.M., Rafelson, N.E., Robert, B., Robert, L. Studies on a human blood platelet protease with elastolytic activity. Biochim. biophys. Acta, _309_, 406, 1973.

18. Marciniak, E., Farley, C.H., De Simone, P.A. Familial thrombosis due to antithrombin III deficiency. Blood, _43_, 219, 1974.

19. Meer, J. van der, Stoepman-van Dalen, E.A., Jansen, J.M.V. Antithrombin III deficiency in a Dutch family. J. Clin. Pathol., _26_, 532, 1973.

20. Moncada, S., Ferreira, S.H., Vane, J.R. Prostaglandins, aspirin-like drugs and the oedema of inflammation. Nature, _246_, 217, 1973.

21. Moore, S. Thrombo-atherosclerosis in normolipemic rabbits: A result of continued endothelial damage. Lab. Invest., _29_, 478, 1973.

22. Moschos, C.B., Lahiri, K., Peter, A., Jesrani, H.N., Regan, T.J. Effect of aspirin upon experimental coronary and non-coronary thrombosis and arrythmia. Am. Heart J., _84_, 525, 1972.

23. Mustard, J.F. Functions of blood platelets and their role in thrombosis. Trans. Am. Clin. Climatol. Assoc., <u>87</u>, 104, 1976.

24. Mustard, J.F., Packman, M.A. The role of blood and platelets in atherosclerosis and the complications of atherosclerosis. Thromb. Diathes. Hemorrh. (Stuttgart), <u>33</u>, 444, 1975.

25. Niewiarowski, S., Regoeczi, E., Stewart, G.J., Senyi, A., Mustard, J.F. Platelet interaction with polymerizing fibrin. J. Clin. Invest., <u>51</u>, 685, 1972.

26. Preston, F.E., Emmanuel, I.G., Winfield, D.A., Malia, R.G. Essential thrombocythemia and peripheral gangrene. Brit. Med. J., <u>3</u>, 548, 1974.

27. Ross, R., Glomset, J.A. The pathogenesis of atherosclerosis. New Engl. J. Med., <u>295</u>, 369, 1976.

28. Ross, R., Harker, L.A. Hyperlipidemia and atherosclerosis. Science, <u>193</u>, 1094, 1976.

29. Ross, R., Glomset, J.A. Atherosclerosis and the smooth muscle cell. Science, <u>180</u>, 1332, 1973.

30. Ross, R., Glomset, J., Kariga, B., Harker, L.A. A platelet-dependent serum factor that stimulates the proliferation of arterial smooth muscle cells in vitro. Proc. Nat. Acad. Sci. USA, <u>71</u>, 1207, 1974.

31. Samuelsson, B., Hamberg, M., Malmsten, C., Svenssen, J. The role of prostaglandin endoperoxides and thrombaxanes in platelet aggregation. Adv. Prostaglandin and Thrombaxane Res., <u>2</u>, 737, 1976. Ed.: B. Samuelsson & R. Paloletti. Raven Press, New York.

32. Silwer, J., Cronberg, S., Nilsson, J.M. Occurrence of arteriosclerosis in von Willebrand's disease. Acta Med. Scand., <u>180</u>, 475, 1966.

33. Smith, J.B., Ingerman, C., Kocsis, J.J., Silver, M.J. Formation of prostaglandins during the aggregation of human blood platelets. J. Clin. Invest., 52, 965, 1973.

34. Steele, P.P., Weily, H.S., Davies, H. and Genton, E. Platelet survival in patients with prosthetic heart valves. New Engl. J. Med., 290, 539, 1974.

35. Stemerman, M.B. Vascular intimal components: precursors of thrombosis. In: Progr. Hemostasis and Thrombosis, 2, 1, 1974. Ed.: T.M. Spaet. Grune & Stratton, New York.

36. Stewart, J.W., Acheson, A.O. Atherosclerosis in a hemophilic. Lancet, 1, 1121, 1957.

37. Vreeken, J., Aken, W.G. van. Spontaneous aggregation of blood platelets as a cause of idiopathic thrombosis and recurrent painful toes and fingers. Lancet, 2, 1394, 1971.

38. Walsh, P.N. Platelet coagulant activities: evidence for multiple different functions of platelets in intrinsic coagulation. Ser. Hemat., 6, 579, 1973.

39. Weily, H.S., Steele , P.P., Davies, H., Pappas, G., Genton, E. Platelet survival in patients with rheumatic heart disease. New Engl. J. Med., 290, 534, 1974.

40. Weiss, H.J. Platelets: Physiology and abnormalities of function. New Engl. J. Med., 293, 531, 1975.

41. Wu, K.K., Hoak, J.C. Spontaneous platelet aggregation in arterial insufficiency: mechanisms and implications. Thromb. Hemostas. (Stuttgart), 35, 702, 1976.

42. Zucker, S., Mielke, C.H. Classification of thrombocytosis based on platelet function tests: correlation with hemorrhagic and thrombotic complications. J. Lab. Clin. Med., 80, 385, 1972.

CHAPTER III
TYPE II^A HYPERLIPOPROTEINEMIA

Meinders, A.E.

Definition: Type II^A hyperlipoproteinemia is a metabolic disorder as a result of genetic defect in the low-density-lipoprotein (L.D.L.) cell-receptor. It is a single gene disorder with an autosomal inheritance pattern. Tendon and tuberous xanthomas and premature coronary artery disease are its main clinical features.

Synonyms: Type II^A hyperlipoproteinemia is also known as familial hyperbetalipoproteinemia, essential familial hypercholesterolemia and hypercholesterolemic familial xanthomatosis.

Detection: Usually little difficulty exists in distinghuishing type II^A pattern from other lipoprotein abnormalities. The presence of hypercholesterolemia with normal plasma triglyceride (T.G.) concentrations is a valuable first step in diagnosis. The plasma will be translucent. The next procedure will be the typing of the lipoprotein pattern. Most of the plasmacholesterol circulates as an intrinsic part of the low - density - lipoprotein (L.D.L.) particle. The reason why the plasma remains clear is the small size of the L.D.L. particles, (22 nm = 220 A). The particles have a core of cholesterol ester and triglyceride and an outer shell of free cholesterol, phospholipids and a pro-

tein called apoprotein B. The percentuel composition is
protein 25%, triglycerides 10%, cholesterol 50% and phospholipids 15%. In the electrophoresis it has beta mobility
and the density is 1019 - 1063. In making the diagnosis
type II^A hyperlipoproteinemia it is of importance to demonstrate increased amounts of LDL or beta lipoproteins in
the plasma. One should however realize that this procedure
is only good for phenotyping patients and might not be
considered as proving a specific genetic lipid disorder.
For this purpose one has to measure cholesterol and triglyceride concentrations in the first degree relatives of
an individual with hyperlipidemia. This offers also the
families the benefit of having younger members with hypercholesterolemia identified before symptomatic disease develops. (In this respect it is of possible importance to
confirm the diagnosis in a child of a known family with
type II^A hyperlipoproteinemia as early as possible. Cord
blood cholesterol determinations have been used and may
improve the probability of a correct diagnosis. Presumably
fibroblast L.D.L. receptor analysis is a more valuable
tool in the future for this purpose).

Another approach, which is not generally available
nowadays but may be so in the future, is demonstrating the
absence (or decreased concentration) of L.D.L. receptorsites in fibroblasts brought in culture. The pathofysiolo-
gical significance of these L.D.L. receptors will be discussed later in this chapter.

It is important to realize that the interpretation
of plasma cholesterol and L.D.L. concentrations is only of
value if the normal distribution of plasma concentrations
in the local population is known. There is a well known

variability not only between populations but also within populations.

In general in the heterozygous state the severity of hypercholesterolemia is variable and may have a range from 300 to more than 500 mg/100 ml. This elevation may, however, exist from early childhood on. In the homozygous state plasma cholesterol concentrations rise above 800 to well over 1000 mg/100 ml with a 4 to 6 times increase of plasma L.D.L. levels. This L.D.L. from type II^A patients is structurally identical to that of normal people. In the general North-American population 1:500 person is a heterozygous carrier of the chromosomal defect. The incidence in post-myocardial infarction patients is much higher and estimated as being 1:20.

Abnormally high plasma L.D.L. concentrations are also found secondary to other diseases (hypothyroidism, porphyria, nefrotic syndrome, autoimmune hyperlipoproteinemia and biliary tract obstruction). Adequate treatment of the primary disorder is followed by restoration of the lipoprotein pattern to normal.

Clinical features

Tendon and Tuberous Xanthomas.

These are yellowish deposits of lipid, which consists for 80% of cholesterol and 90% of this cholesterol is esterified with oleic acid. It is generally thought that the cholesterol in the lesions originates from plasma and is not locally synthesized. Labelled cholesterol and labelled L.D.L. injected intravenously enter the xanthomas and no cholesterol is formed from i.v. administered labelled acetate.

Tendon xanthomas are found predominantly in the
Achilles tendons and the extensor tendons of the hands.
They may, however, also be detected in the tendons of the
extensor muscles of the foot, peroneus muscle, in the plan-
tar aponeurosis and subperiostally below the knees and
the olecranon proces. The tendinous lesions in the hands
occasionally cause distortion and erosion of the finger
joints.

Tuberous xanthomas are found intra- and subcutaneous-
ly. They are flat, slightly raised, planar lesions and
tend to be distributed over the buttocks, thighs, elbows,
knees and webs of fingers.

Xanthomas are seen in homozygous and heterozygous
patients. Generally they appear earlier in life in the
homozygous persons, who may even be born with them. Usually they are present before the age of 20 years. In heterozygous patients they become manifest between 30 and 60
years. Supposedly the presence or absence of xanthomas
depends on the degree as well as the duration of the hypercholesterolemia.

Xanthomas form no complete proof of type II^A hyperlipoproteinemia as they are also seen in secondary hypercholesterolemia and also in type III hyperlipoproteinemia.

Xanthelasmata.

This yellowish intracutaneous lipid deposition around
the eyes, is less specific for the diagnosis of type II^A
hyperlipoproteinemia as they can be seen in other disturbances of lipid metabolism and also in persons with normal
blood lipid levels. Patients with type II^A hyperlipoproteinemia with tendon xanthomas have in over 70% xanthelasmata.

Corneal Arcus.

This yellow-white corneal ring consists of cholesterol, triglycerides and phospholipids and is a common finding in normal elderly people. If discovered before the age of 40 years it might be a symptom of type II^A hyperlipoproteinemia.

Hyperuricemia and cholesterolstones don't seem to be related to type II^A hypercholesterolemia.

Arthritis.

Transient attacks of arthritis, affecting mostly the knees, ankles and hands and lasting a few days occur in about half the homozygote patients. The affected joints become inflamed, swollen and painful and fever may exist during the attack. No cause is known for this clinical feature. The arthritis is seen in patients with tendinous xanthomas.

Cardiovascular disease

Atherosclerosis is a prominent feature of type II^A hyperlipoproteinemia. The very extensive atheromatous degeneration is biochemically not different from the same lesions found in the normal aging population. The atherosclerotic plaques are predominantly situated in the coronary arteries and the abdominal aorta in the heterozygotes, while in the homozygotes the aortic valves and the ascending aorta are also involved. Homozygotes usually die from myocardial infarction before the age of 30 years. Heterozygotes females have a mean age of 60 years and males of 50 years at the time of dying, usually from myocardial infarction. Clinically peripheral arterial vascular disease is of much less importance in type II^A hyperlipoproteinemia. This is true for cerebrovascular disease and obliterating vascular disease of the extremities.

In asymptomatic patients a systolic heart murmur and ischemic electrocardiographic changes may be found after exercise or even in rest.

In general most studies agree that type II^A lipoproteinemia makes a significant contribution to the incidence of ischemic heart disease in the general population, although there is disagreement as to the extent of this contribution. In a group of patients with myocardial infarction 2% of the males and 5% of the females was diagnosed via family studies as having type II^A hyperlipoproteinemia. This incidence was higher among patients below the age of 55 years.

Genetics.

Type II^A hyperlipoproteinemia has an autosomal dominant inheritance pattern. There is a single gene locus mutation. The expression of the disease is more marked in patients with two copies of the gene than with a single copy. The plasma cholesterol concentration in homozygotes is approximately twice that in heterozygotes and about four times that in the normal local population.

In some areas in the world the frequency of heterozygotes is very high. In Libanon it is as high as 1 to 80. The prolonged survival of the mutant gene is in accordance with the fact that its effect on genetic fitness in the heterozygote is small and that most heterozygotes become old enough to have children.

The genetic disorder of type II^A hyperlipoproteinemia may, sometimes in the same family, have a different phenotype, as shown by the occurrence of type II^B hyperlipoproteinemia, in some members of the family.

It is clear that genetic counselling of the families with known type II^A hyperlipoproteinemia is of the utmost importance and that detection of homozygous offspring at the earliest opportunity might be of value for starting treatment.

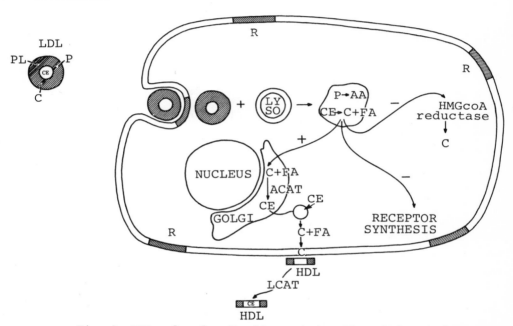

Fig. 1 LDL = low density lipoprotein, CE = cholesterolesters, C = cholesterol, P = protein, PL = phospholipid, R = Receptorsite, Lyso = lysosome, AA = Amino-acids, FA = fatty-acids, ACAT = acylCoA-cholesterol-acyl transferase, LCAT = lecithine-cholesterol-acyl transferase, HDL = high density lipoprotein, HMG = hydroxy-methyl-glutaraat.

Pathophysiology. (Figure 1)

Cultured fibroblasts from normal as well as type II^A

hyperlipoproteinemic patients are able to synthesize cholesterol as do hepatocytes. Studies with these fibroblasts have thrown much light on the cellular mechanism of this lipid disorder.

Normally the L.D.L. cholesterol particles are bound to a cellreceptor of high affinity and specifity. By endocytosis L.D.L. is internalized and fusion occurs with lysosomes. A breakdown of the lipoprotein structure occurs and the protein fraction is destructed by proteases. The cholesterol ester is hydrolysed and free cholesterol enters the extralysosomal cellular compartment. This unesterified cholesterol regulates three intracellular events: suppression of 3 - hydroxy - 3 methyl - glutaryl coenzyme A reductase, which catalizes the production of mevalonic acid, a precursor in cholesterol synthesis; induction of another enzyme cholesteryl acyl transferase, which causes reesterification of cholesterol and storage of the cholesterol esters; feedback suppression of L.D.L. receptorsites, preventing excessive accumulation of cholesterol. The defect in type II^A hyperlipoproteinemia is the complete or incomplete absence of L.D.L. receptorsites. Homozygotes have receptor - negative cells and in heterozygotes the amount of the L.D.L. receptorsites is reduced by 50%. A second type of mutation has been found in which receptor - defective cells exist with about 10% of the normal amount of L.D.L. receptorsites. It is of interest to know that these patients react favourably to conventional therapy compared to the receptor-negative homozygotes.

The total absence of receptorsites in the homozygotes results in an enormous increase (60 x) of the rate controlling enzyme 3 H-3MG Co A reductase intracellularly and consequently an increased cholesterol production in the presence of already elevated plasma cholesterol levels.

There is a threefold reduction of L.D.L. catabolism and a twofold to threefold overproduction of L.D.L. In heterozygotes, with 50% reduction in L.D.L. receptors the production of cholesterol and the production and degradation of L.D.L. is normal but at the expence of a twofold to threefold elevation of plasma L.D.L. concentrations.

Therapy

See chapter on therapy of lipid disorders. (XIX)

Literature

1. Breslow, J.L., et al. (1975): New Engl. J. Med., 293, 900.
2. Brown, M.S., et al. (1976): New Engl. J. Med., 294, 1386.
3. DeWitt, S. Goodman (1976): In: The Year in Metabolism, p. 153.
4. Myant, N.B., et al. (1973): Clinics in Endocrinology and Metabolism, 2, 81.
5. Schade, R.W.B. (1976): Thesis. University of Nijmegen.
6. Small, D.M. (1977): New Engl. J. Med., 297, 873.

CHAPTER IV

HYPERLIPOPROTEINEMIA, METABOLISM OF TRIGLYCERIDES

Sailer, S.

Besides cholesterol, triglycerides are regarded as a major risk factor for the development of atherosclerosis. Therefore, many studies have been carried out during the last years in order to clarify the pathomechanisms which lead to hypertriglyceridemia.

1. Normal metabolism of free fatty acids (F.F.A.) and triglycerides (T.G.)

The F.F.A. are long chain fatty acids which serve as an important source of calories for many tissues of the body during periods of fasting. They are transported between adipose tissue and other tissues using plasma albumin as a vehicle. The concentration of F.F.A. in the plasma is very low (20 mg%), but the F.F.A. turnover is very high. F.F.A. are taken up by many tissues, but a large fraction is removed by the liver, where the F.F.A. may be oxidized or incorporated into T.G. of very low density lipoproteins (V.L.D.L.). The fraction which gives rise to T.G. in V.L.D.L. is under nutritional control: It is higher after a carbohydrate rich diet than during a period of fasting. Of course, the net uptake of F.F.A. by the liver is determined by the concentration of F.F.A. in the blood and thus regulates also the secretion rate of T.G. as V.L.D.L.-T.G. from the liver.

The liver produces V.L.D.L. primarily from endogenous sources of lipids. The intestinal mucosa is responsible for the production of chylomicrons and V.L.D.L. primarily from exogenous or dietary lipids absorbed from the intestinal lumen. In man, the *de novo* synthesis of lipids from glucose seem to play a minor role.

Once these nascent lipoproteins enter the circulation, assimilation of T.G. contained in chylomicrons and V.L.D.L. is a complex interacting between these lipoprotein particles and the enzyme lipoprotein lipase which is located on capillary endothelial surface. This enzyme hydrolyzes T.G. to F.F.A., partial glycerides and glycerol. The lipids are taken up partly by the tissue cells, the glycerol appears in the blood stream. Of particular interest is the obligatory role of phospholipids and an apolipoprotein cofactor for triglyceride hydrolysis by adipose tissue lipoprotein lipase. This protein cofactor, identified as apolipoprotein glutamic acid (ApoC$_{II}$) is abundant in the high density lipoprotein (H.D.L.) fraction of plasma lipoproteins. It was shown, that this cofactor necessary for the breakdown of T.G.-rich lipoproteins is transferred from H.D.L. to the chylomicrons and V.L.D.L. immediately if these particles enter the circulation in "nascent" form. By this process, the T.G. in chylomicrons and V.L.D.L. become an activated substrate necessary for the activity of lipoprotein lipase. These activated T.G.-rich particles passing the capillary bed are catabolized by the action of lipoprotein lipase: The T.G. are hydrolyzed forming F.F.A. and glycerol, thus the particles

become smaller, the T.G. content decreases, the relative
cholesterol content increases, the density of these newly
formed particles is higher. Finally the activator apoprotein C_{II} is retransferred to the H.D.L. fraction. By
the process particles are formed which are poor in T.G.
content, contain only traces of apoprotein C, contain
still the apoprotein B, the cholesterol content is high,
the density increases, the migration rate in the electric
field is slower (β-Band) than that of V.L.D.L.: Low
density lipoproteins (L.D.L.) and/or "remnants" are
formed.

2. *T.G. Metabolism in hyperlipoproteinemia*

The insight into the mechanism governing normal
lipoproteins metabolism now make it easier to understand
the pathophysiology behind the hyperlipoproteinemias.
a) *Type I* (Familial hyperchylomicronemia, fat induced
    hyperlipidemia, familial exogenous hypertriglyceridemia)
This disease is characterized by a marked elevation
of T.G.-rich chylomicrons even in fasting plasma. While
the patient is on a normal diet, the plasma T.G./choleste-
rol ratio may exceed 10. When these patients are placed
on a fat free diet the chylomicrons disappear within a
few days. Clinical findings include episodic abdominal
pain, hepatosplenomegaly, eruptive xanthomas, and pancreatitis apparently caused by the lipemia. An active
lipoprotein lipase is not present to a significant extent
in post-heparin plasma in type I patients, nor does there
appear to be lipoprotein lipase activity in adipose tissue
of affected individuals. Therefore, the molecular defect
in type I hyperlipoproteinemia lies in the enzyme lipoprotein lipase, *per se* or in one of the steps leading to

its synthesis. The prognosis is not normal because of recurrent pancreatitis, but they do not seem to be prone to atherosclerosis.

b) *Type III* (Broad β-disease, remnant disease, dyslipoproteinemia).

This disease is characterized by an increased concentration of T.G. and of cholesterol in the plasma, as a result of the presence of an unusual class of lipoproteins of a density of d 1.019 g/ml and a relatively high proportion of an arginine-rich apolipoprotein. It can be regarded as an "abnormal T.G.-rich L.D.L.". Electrophoresis of whole plasma usually shows a single broad band which extends from the β into the pre-β region. Chylomicrons are sometimes visible. The incidence of premature vascular disease in type III hyperlipoproteinemia is high.

Because of the metabolic relationships of the V.L.D.L. as a precursor to L.D.L., and the chemical and physical properties of the "abnormal" lipoprotein of type III, the observation has been made that this lipoprotein may be a "remnant" of V.L.D.L. catabolism for which T.G. removal is incomplete. It is uncertain whether it is an abnormal lipoprotein or an abnormal accumulation of an intermediate of lipoprotein metabolism.

The familial nature of type III seems firmly established, but the mode of inheritance is presently unexplained. only recently a defect in an apolipoprotein (E_{III}) in these patients was detected. This defect could explain easily the disturbed catabolism of V.L.D.L. in these patients.

c) *Type IV* (Hyperpre-β-lipoproteinemia, familial hyperlipemia, carbohydrate-induced hyperlipemia, endogenous hyperlipemia).

Type IV is characterized by an elevation in concentration during fasting of plasma V.L.D.L. or pre-β-lipoproteins. Since these lipoproteins are T.G.-rich, plasma T.G. are elevated. Premature coronary artery disease is very frequent (about 50% of the patients).

Type IV does not seem to be a nosological entity. This makes interpretation of data concerning the metabolic defect of this type very difficult. In spite of the fact, that the lipoprotein lipase system seems to be normal in these patients, in most cases decreased rates of catabolism of V.L.D.L. were demonstrated. An increased F.F.A. supply to the liver or an increased rate of lipogenesis in the liver seems not to play a significant role in the pathogenesis of this disease.

d) *Type V* (Familial mixed (endogenous and exogenous) hyperlipemia)).

In type V elevated levels of V.L.D.L. and chylomicrons are found in fasting plasma. Chronic pancreatitis is often present and severe acute attacks may occur. The incidence of coronary heart disease is not very high in these patients. Alcohol may be a pathogenetic factor, but the biochemical defect is not understood. Clearance of dietary fat is impaired, and post-heparin lipolytic activity may be low. The transmission of the genetic defect is unclear.

CHAPTER V

ATHEROSCLEROSIS IN THYROIDAL AND ADRENAL DISEASES

Doorenbos, H.

Atherosclerosis may be defined as a condition in which generalized vascular damage is present with atheroma formation in the main arteries resulting in their partial occlusion and diminished blood flow. It is caused by a number of factors, including vascular injury for example by hypertension and elevation of the cholesterol and possibly also triglyceride content of blood. Clinical symptoms appear only when the circulation is either severely compromised already or when heavy demands are made upon it. It is not intended to give here a survey of the influence of thyroid hormone on lipid metabolism. In general it may be said, that it increases both lipolysis and triglyceride synthesis and increases synthesis of cholesterol while lowering its plasma concentration. Thyroid disease affects the circulation both in conditions with thyroid hormone excess and in hypothyroidism. As in myxedema the overall metabolism has slowed down considerably, the extent to which bloodflow is compromised will become clinically evident only after treatment with thyroid hormone has begun. In thyrotoxicosis all organ systems of the body are functioning at a high level, cardiac output is high and peripheral resistence low as the small blood vessels are dilated because of the high oxygen consumption and the loss of heat in the periphery. Pulse-pressure is high. Energy intake and output are markedly

increased. This does not imply that the cholesterol and
triglyceride content of the blood are normal or low. Nowadays overweight does not exclude the diagnosis of hyperthyroidism, nor does hypercholesterolemia or hypertriglyceridemia. The latter may be caused by coexisting diabetes mellitus or excessive use of alcohol. Following treatment of
the thyrotoxicosis it is to be expected that the diastolic
bloodpressure rises somewhat, though seldom in the pathological range. The course of the disturbance of carbohydrate intolerance when present, depends more on what happens
with body weight, than on the thyroid hormone content of
the blood. This also applies to the lipid components in
the serum, at least for the time euthyroidism does not pass
into hypothyroidism.

When part of the thyroid is ablated i.e. either by
surgery or by treatment with radioactive iodine,myxedema
occurs in a high percentage of cases. Two forms may be
distinghuished. The so called early myxedema is apparent
within 3 months after treatment when too large a part of the
thyroid has been ablated. The late myxedema presents itself in a higher percentage every year following ablative
therapy,affecting ultimately between 40-80% of cases and
has a very insidious onset. It is thought to be due to continuing destruction of thyroid hormone producing tissue
by thyroiditis of autoimmune origin.

Many of the clinical signs of atherosclerosis are
mirrored by incipient hypothyroidism. Therefore the question
is relevant whether diminished thyroid function causes
atherosclerosis. It has been stated that overt hypothyroidism is associated with an increased incidence of ischaemic heart disease. Moreover in subclinical hypothyroidism
as defined by the presence of thyroid antibodies and lympho-

cytic infiltration of the thyroid a raised serumcholesterol
and ischaemic heart disease were seen more often. In an
epidemiological survey it was found that there is a significant association between subclinical hypothyroidism
as characterized by elevated serum TSH and minor ECG changes
in the female,using the Minnesota code after exclusion of
other known risk factors. This was not found in the male.
Nor was there any association between the presence of antibodies and ECG changes in either sex after elimination of
other risk factors. It should also be remembered, that a
repolarisation disturbance in overt hypothyroidism need
not be indicative of occlusive coronary disease, as it may
disappear within a few weeks after proper thyroid hormone
replacement therapy has been given.

Recently the results of an epidemiological study have
been published concerning the frequency of thyroid disease
and blood lipid abnormalities in 2700 people. Overt and
possible hyperthyroidism were found in 19 resp.29 per thousand
females and 1.6 resp. 2.3 per thousand males. Overt and possible
hypothyroidism were seen in 14 resp. 19 per thousand females and
less than one per thousand males. In this population sample
there was no relation between thyroid dysfunction and abnormalities in blood lipid pattern. Even so, when the
decision is made to treat hyperlipidaemia,   the possible
existence of hypothyroidism should always be excluded and
when present this condition should be treated first.

Hypothyroidism may be either primary or secondary.
Secondary hypothyroidism is caused by pathology in the
hypothalamic/pituitary region. Its clinical picture depends
on the presence or absence of signs of increased intra-
cranial pressure and even more on the functional capacity
of the pituitary to secrete ACTH and gonadotropins. In

general it can be said that hypopituitary patients with approximately normal ACTH production are normal – or over-weight, while those with deficient ACTH production are underweight. In secondary hypothyroidism there may be hyperlipidemia but it is usually of lesser degree than when the thyroid itself is the cause of the myxedema.

Primary hypothyroidism usually is the endpoint of autoimmune thyroiditis. It may be accelerated by previous ablative therapy. Thyroid dysfunction may be accentuated in unfavourable circumstances e.g. exposure to iodine excess, goitrogenic substances or treatment of psychiatric disease with lithiumcarbonate. Laboratory diagnosis of thyroid insufficiency uses determinations of TSH, serum thyroxin and the free thyroxin index. Tracer studies with radioactive iodine do not give the necessary information nor does the determination of T3. A TRH test is usually not required, except in cases with hypothalamic/pituitary disturbance, and here the data obtained are often ambiguous. All tests may give misleading results when not performed under proper conditions.

Elevation of TSH is seen in a number of conditions not indicative of primary hypothyroidism. Yet it is the single most sensitive laboratory sign of this condition. When absent, primary hypothyroidism can confidently be excluded as the cause of the presenting signs of atherosclerosis. When present, thyroid dysfunction should not be accepted unquestioningly as the cause of the patient's complaints. When secondary hypothyroidism is suspected, TSH determinations and even TRH tests will not be of sufficient help in diagnosis. Usually a low serum thyroxin in the presence of other signs of endocrine insufficiency and local pituitary pathology will point in the right direction.

The preferred treatment of hypothyroidism nowadays is thyroxin given in increasing doses with increments every week while regularly repeating ECG's. If the coronary condition permits, a full substitution dose is reached in 6-8 weeks, being 150-200 ug for the 70 kg individual. The time is not long past that patients were being made hypothyroid on purpose to treat their crippling angina. We have never used this mode of therapy, but have on occasion abstained from giving thyroid hormone to patients with severe coronary insufficiency. The outcome in them has been uniformly disastrous after a short interval. Therefore we believe that thyroid hormone substitution should be pushed as high as the subjective and objective signs will permit, even though this implies the occasional occurrence of a therapy induced myocardial infarction.

Of the adrenal cortical hormones in man cortisol is the most important one influencing lipid metabolism. In as much as dysfunction of the adrenal cortex plays a role in causing hypertension this may be an additive factor in the etiology of atherosclerotic vascular disease. Cortisol has a protein wasting activity, inhibiting aminoacid uptake in cells, increasing gluconeogenesis in the liver and suppressing growth hormone release and effect. It increases appetite. Insuline resistance occurs with mild diabetes. Synthesis of fat is increased, being deposited in the localisation typical for Cushing's syndrome. Untreated Cushing's syndrome results in death within 5 years in about 50% of cases from infection or from atherosclerotic vascular disease.

The cause of Cushing's syndrome may be overproduction of pituitary ACTH, an adrenal adenoma or carcinoma, ectopic

ACTH production and iatrogenic, following treatment with cortisol analogues. In cases of ectopic ACTH production the decline in overall condition caused by the hormone producing malignancy is so rapid, that atherosclerotic complications do not play a major part in the final outcome. The same is the case in patients with adrenal carcinoma, where progress of the disease may be so rapid, that the classical symptoms of Cushing's syndrome are not given time to develop. In iatrogenic hypercorticism the course of the underlying disease for which steroids are being given is the main determinant whether atherosclerotic complications will present themselves. In the early days when steroids were being given indiscriminately for relatively benign conditions thromboembolism and myocardial infarction where frequently seen. Nowadays even though sometimes extremely high doses are being used for prolonged periods as in severe blood dyscrasias or following transplantation, supervening therapy-resistent infection has taken first place as the cause of death in iatrogenic Cushing's syndrome.

The diagnosis of hypercorticism caused by hypersecretion of ACTH or by an adrenal adenoma, both conditions that develop insidiously, can be made using low and high dose dexamethasone suppression tests. Determination of the cortisol secretion rate may also be of value, but difficulties in interpretation may arise when correction should be made for overweight. In the out-patient clinic the short dexamethasone suppression test giving 1 mg at 23 hrs on the night preceding the early morning cortisol determination has proved its value as a screening test. When the diagnosis has been firmly established, therapy should consist of surgical ablation of part of the adrenal tissue, total adrenalectomy or/and measures against pituitary dysfunction as indicated.

In conclusion the most important endocrine disorder causing accelerated atherosclerosis is primary hypothyroidism. Cushing's syndrome due to overproduction of ACTH or adrenal adenoma ranks second place, while iatrogenic Cushing's syndrome is not of as much importance as it used to be since steroids are being used less indiscriminately.

Literature

1. Bakker, K. (1977): The influence of lithiumcarbonate on the hypothalamic pituitary thyroid axis. MD Thesis, Groningen.
2. Bastenie, P.A., Bonnyns, M., Vanhaelst, L., Neve, P. and Staquet, M. (1971): Preclinical hypothyroidism, a risk factor for coronary heart disease. Lancet I, 203.
3. Baxter, J.D. and Forsham, P.H. (1972): Tissue effects of glucocorticoids. Am. J. Med. 53, 573.
4. Braverman, I.E., Woeber, K.E. and Ingbar S.H. (1969): Induction of myxedema by iodine in patients euthyroid after radioiodine or surgical treatment of diffuse toxic goiter. New Engl. J. Med. 281, 816.
5. Burden, A.C., Rosenthal, F.D. and Swales J.D. (1977): Sodium metabolism, plasmarenin and thyroid hormone deficiency. Clin. Sc. Mol. Med. 53, 3.
6. Lange, W.E. de, Reitsma, W.D. Visser, J.W.E. and Doorenbos, H. (1969): The effect of treatment of hyperthyroidism and myxoedema on glucose assimilation and the response of free fatty acids and insulin after intravenous administration of glucose. Ned. T. v. Geneesk. 113, 649.
7. Editorial (1971): Therapeutic possibilities in Cushing's syndrome. New Engl. J. Med. 285, 288.

8. Fowler, P.B.S. and Swale, J. (1970): Hypercholesterolemia in borderline hypothyroidism. Lancet 2, 488.

9. Fowler, P.B.S. and Swale, J. (1967): Premyxedema and coronary artery disease. Lancet 1, 1077.

10. Gordin, A., Saarinen, P., Pelkonen, R. and Lamberg, B.A. (1974): Serum thyrotrophin and the response to TRH in symptomless autoimmune thyroiditis and in borderline and overt hypothyroidism. Acta Endocr. 75, 274.

11. Heinonen, O.P., Aro, K., Pyörälä, et al. (1972): Symptomless autoimmune thyroiditis in coronary heart disease. Lancet 1, 785.

12. Kersen, F. van (1973): TRH, TSH en schildklierfunctie. MD Thesis, Groningen (Dutch).

13. Lamberts, S.W.J. and Birkenhäger, J.C. (1976): Body composition in Cushing's syndrome. J. Clin. Endocr. Met. 42, 864.

14. Lamberg, B.A. (1965): Glucose metabolism in thyroid disease. Acta Med. Scand. 178, 351.

15. Miettinen, T.A. (1968): Mechanism of serum cholesterol reduction by thyroid hormones in hypothyroidism. J. Lab. Clin. Med. 71, 539.

16. Nerup, J. and Binder, C. (1973): Thyroid, gastric and adrenal autoimmunity in diabetes mellitus. Acta Endocr. 72, 279.

17. Nichols, T., Nugent, C.A. and Tyler, F.H. (1968): Steroid laboratory tests in the diagnosis of Cushing's syndrome. Am. J. Med. 45, 116.

18. Nugent, C.A., Nichols, T. and Tyler, F.H. (1965): Diagnosis of Cushing's syndrome - single dose dexamethasone suppression test. Arch. Int. Med. 116, 172.

19. Palmblad, J., Levi, J., Burger, A., Melander, A. et al. (1977): Effects of fasting on the levels of growth

hormone, thyrotropin, cortisol, adrenaline, noradre-
naline, T4, T3 and rT3 in healthy males. Acta Med.
Scand. 201, 15.

20. Patel, Y.L. and Burger, H.G. (1973): Serum TSH in pituitary and/or hypothalamic hypothyroidism: normal or
elevated basal levels and paradoxical responses to
thyrotropin releasing hormone. J. Clin. Endocr. 37,
190.

21. Porte, D., Graber, A.L. et al. (1966): The effect of
epinephrine on immunoreactive insulin levels in man.
J. Clin. Invest. 45, 228.

22. Toft, A.D., Boyns, A.R., Cole, E.N. et al. (1973): The
effect of TRH on plasma prolactin and thyrotropin levels
in primary hypothyroidism. Clin. Endocr. 2, 289.

23. Toft, A.D., Irvine, W.J., Hunter, W.M., Rathcliffe,
J.G. and Seth, J. (1974): Anomalous plasma TSH levels
in patients developing hypothyroidism in the early
months after ^{131}J therapy for thyrotoxicosis. J. Clin.
Endocr. Met. 39, 607.

24. Tulloch, B.R., Lewis, B. and Russel Fraser, T. (1973):
Triglyceride metabolism in thyroid disease. Lancet 1,
391.

25. Tunbridge, W.M.G., Evered, D.C., Hall, R. et al. (1977):
Lipid profiles and cardiovascular disease in the Whick-
ham area with particular reference to thyroid failure.
Clin. Endocr. 7, 495.

26. Tunbridge, W.M.G., Evered, D.C., Hall, R. et al. (1977): The
spectrum of thyroid disease in a community. Clin. Endocr.
7, 481.

27. Vanhaelst, L., Neve, P., Chailly, P. and Bastenie, P.A.
(1967): Coronary artery disease in hypothyroidism.
Lancet 2, 800.

CHAPTER VI
GONADAL HORMONES AND ATHEROSCLEROSIS

Reitsma, W.D.

Our present knowledge on the biochemical and metabolic effects of gonadal hormones is for the greater part based on the numerous publications on the effects of contraceptive steroids. Birth control pills essentially consist of a combination of an estrogenic component and a progestational agent. The estrogen components are either ethinyl estradiol or its 3-methyl ether mestranol. The progestational agents are derived from two basic groups: 19 nortestosterones and 17αhydroxyprogesterone derivatives. A workshop on the effects of gonadal hormones and contraceptives held in Boston almost ten years ago has been a great stimulus for further research and forms the basis of our present understanding of many side effects of gonadal hormones. (Salhanick e.a. 1969). Surveying the literature with respect to a possible relationship between gonadal hormones and atherosclerosis, the following effects of gonadal hormones should be discussed: modifications of carbohydrate and lipid metabolism, alterations which may result in hypertension and interaction with blood coagulation.

Carbohydrate metabolism

In healthy young women the use of the oral contra-

ceptive Lyndiol$^{(R)}$, a combination of mestranol and lynestrenol, a nortestosterone derivative, induces a rise of
the glucose level after overnight fasting and in the course of a glucose tolerance test. Insulin levels also increase. (Terpstra 1971). These alterations are more pronounced after a longer period of treatment. Withdrawal of
the oral contraceptive results already after one month in
an improvement of the glucose tolerance.

The separate administration of either synthetic
estrogens or progesterone derivatives does not consistent-
ly alter glucose or insulin levels. (Beck 1973). Only a
large single injection of a depot preparation of medroxy-
progesterone acetate induces a slight deterioration of the
glucose tolerance with concurrent increases of plasma insulin concentrations. Nortestosterone derivatives, however, like norethindrone given in sufficiently high doses
produce a deterioration in glucose tolerance. In birth
control pills the estrogenic component appears to potentiate the hyperglycemic effect of nortestosterone derivatives. Contraceptives, that contain a nortestosterone
derivative like ethynodiol diacetate, lynestrenol and norethindrone, give a higher incidence of decreased glucose
tolerance than pills that contain a progesterone derivative like chloormadinone acetate.

The alterations in carbohydrate metabolism, which are
induced by oral contraceptives in normal women are slight.
The one hour postglucose concentration shifts only 10-20
mg/dl upward. After withdrawal of the contraceptive glucose tolerance improves again. The data on the effect of
oral contraceptives in women with a decreased ability to
secrete insulin are scarce. A more pronounced effect on
glucose levels, however, is to be expected. In patients

with latent diabetes and possibly also in prediabetes this results in a higher incidence of a deterioration in glucose tolerance. Therefore one should use some restraint in prescribing oral contraceptives to women with latent diabetes or a pronounced family history of diabetes. In patients, however, who use insulin for treatment of their diabetes mellitus, daily insulin requirement does not significantly increase under the influence of oral contraceptives. Therefore there is no special reason to refuse to women with manifest diabetes, treated with insulin, the use of oral contraceptives.

Lipid metabolism

In women with intact ovaries serum cholesterol levels increase with age. In young women oophorectomy leads to an increase in circulating cholesterol, but not in women over 45. Mestranol lowers cholesterol in early oophorectomized women. In postmenopausal women estrogens increase H.D.L.-cholesterol but lower L.D.L.-cholesterol. Nortestosterone derivatives seem to counteract the effect of synthetic estrogens. Increasing doses of norethindrone are associated with increasing fasting cholesterol levels at a constant dose of estrogen. The administration of Lyndiol has according to our own experience in healthy young women little or no effect on serum cholesterol levels.

Estrogen and estrogen containing contraceptives increase serum T.G. (triglyceride) levels of normal women. The mechanism by which estrogens elevate serum T.G. is still not entirely clear. Increased hepatic production of T.G. is probably the most important factor. The positive association between a rise of serum gamma glutamyl transpeptidase activity and triglyceride concentration during oral contraceptive therapy may reflect hepatic microsomal enzyme induction (Martin e.a. 1976). The rise of T.G. appears predominantly in the low density lipoprotein fraction which is presumed to be synthesized in the liver.

On the other hand also a decrease of the plasma clearing rate of T.G. may play a role. Estrogens depress plasma heparin like activity (P.H.L.A.). P.H.L.A. consists of two activities: hepatic T.G. lipase and extrahepatic lipoprotein lipase. The decrease of P.H.L.A. is caused by a selective decline of hepatic triglyceride lipase. The change of hepatic triglyceride lipase during estrogen therapy, however, does not correlate with the increase in triglycerides (Applebaum e.a. 1977). A reduction of P.H.L.A. to approximately 50% has also been shown during longterm estrogen-progestagen treatment.

Nortestosterone derivatives like norethindrone lower T.G. in many subjects. No changes were observed with progesterone. Birth control pill combinations containing progesterone derivatives generally produce a more marked rise in T.G. than those containing nortestosterone derivatives. In our own experience Lyndiol induces after three month treatment a small but significant rise in serum T.G. (Terpstra 1971). The finding that contraceptive steroids like estrogens produce a rise in triglycerides without inducing hyperglycemia may represent a shunting of glucose in the liver from gluconeogenic pathways to triglyceride synthesizing pathways. In rat livers such an effect has been demonstrated, estradiol benzoate and progesterone inhibiting gluconeogenesis. The effect of combined contraceptive steroids on serum glucose and T.G. will be the resultant of the effects of both components and their interaction. Possibly estrogens inhibit the biliary excretion of nortestosterone derivatives and slow their excretion.

The effect of contraceptive administration may also depend from the metabolic state of the patient receiving treatment. In obese women triglyceride levels generally increase to the same degree (about 20%) as in normal women. The results in patients with hyperlipoproteinemia are equivocal. Birth control pill may grossly exaggarate hypertriglyceridemia in type IV hyperlipoproteinemia. On the other hand therapy with estrogens may correct hyper-lipemia in type III hypertriglyceridemia in despite of an increase of T.G.-production, by correction of the impaired catabolism of very low density lipoproteins (Chait e.a. 1977).

The increased frequency of the occurrence of gall-stones in women using oral contraceptives probably re-flects the alterations of lipid metabolism. Oral contra-ceptives decrease the proportion of chenodeoxycholic acid while increasing the cholesterol saturation of bile (Ben-nion e.a. 1976). This makes the bile more lithogenic. The relation between oral contraceptives to gallbladder disease is not surprising. It is consistent with the known higher rates of gallbladder disease among women as compared with man.

Renin-angiotensin-aldosterone system

During pregnancy and to a lesser degree during the second half of the menstrual cycle are both plasma renin activity (P.R.A.) and aldosterone levels increased. Estro-gens induce an increase in plasma renin substrate (P.R.S.) and P.R.A. (Katz and Beck 1974). Progesterone is an al-dosterone antagonist and the resulting natriuresis is

64

thought to induce a compensatory increase in renin secretion. The combination estrogen-progestogen contraceptives also elevate P.R.S. and P.R.A. but plasma aldosterone is not significantly altered by these agents.
Hyperaldosteronism therefore cannot explain the occurrence
of hypertension in about 5% of the women using birth control pills. Moreover hypokaliemie is not found in oral
contraceptive hypertension.

Recent studies demonstrated a reduction of renal flow
and an inappropriate rise in circulating angiotensine II
concentration for the state of sodium balance during the
use of oral contraceptives (Hollenberg e.a. 1976). The
inability to neutralize the increase in P.R.S., which
occurs in every women using contraceptive steroids, is
generally thought to cause oral contraceptive hypertension.
The presence, however, of histologically demonstrable abnormalities in peripheral renal vessels like microthrombi
has also been demonstrated in patients who develop hypertension while taking estrogen progestogen containing compounds (Boyd e.a. 1975). The arise of hypertension during
oral contraceptive treatment forms a reason to withdraw
the drug. If this does not result in a normalisation of
the blood pressure within three months further investigation is needed.

Bloodcoagulation
There is a striking rise in the incidence of venous
thrombosis and pulmonary embolism in women using contraceptives as compared with women of the same age. In older
women above 35 years of age a six to sevenfold increase
has been reported, while in younger women the risk of
thromboembolism was two times higher in pill users. It is

likely that changes in the clotting mechanism contribute
to the thrombotic tendency in women on contraceptives.
During oral contraceptive treatment there is a decrease of
antithrombin III activity, which has an important function
to neutralize activated clotting factors II, VII, IX, X
and XI. There is a temporary increase of the fibrinogen
level. Though there is an increase in the potential for
fibrin formation, also increased fibrinolytic activity
has been reported (Hedlin 1975). Generally there will
therefore be a tendency to maintain a balance between the
two systems. However, it is not surprising that this
balance may become seriously disturbed in some women resulting in thromboembolic complications.

    There are many indications that neutral female sex
hormones protect against atherosclerotic alterations. The
incidence of coronary heart disease in man below fifty
years of age is five times higher as compared with women
of the same age. High density lipoproteins, which possibly
protect against atherosclerosis are lower in man than in
women. In women, whose menopause is premature, an increased
prevalence of coronary heart disease has been reported.
    There is a strong evidence, that synthetic sex ste-
roids may have an opposite effect. Elderly males treated
with stilbestrol because of prostatic carcinoma show an
increased incidence of myocardial infarction. Though oral
contraceptives induce only a small rise of blood glucose
and triglyceride levels, and result only sometimes in a
reversible hypertension, the risk of myocardial infarction
is increased. Epidemiological studies revealed an increased cardiovascular mortality rate of three to five

times associated with the use of contraceptive steroids
(Beral 1976, Ory 1977). This holds true especially for
women 40 years of age or older. (Mann e.a. 1975). In
women over 40 and if other risk factors exist such as
heavy cigarette smoking, hypertension and hypercholesterolemia, alternative methods of contraception like intra
uterine device (I.U.D.) and sterilisation should be considered. (Hennekens and MacMahon 1977).

Summarizing we may come to the following conclusions:

1) Overt diabetes mellitus is not a reason to abstain from
   the use of oral contraceptives. In latent diabetes
   there is probably an increased risk of the development
   of manifest diabetes.
2) The arise of hypertension or thromboembolic complications during oral contraceptive treatment is a reason
   to stop the contraceptive and prescribe an other method
   of contraception.
3) The risk of myocardial infarction attributable to oral
   contraceptives seems to be greatest in women over 40.
   In this group alternative methods of contraception
   should be encouraged.

Literature

1) Applebaum, D.M., Goldberg, A.P., Pikälisto, A.J., Brunzell, J.D. and Hazzard, W.R. (1977): Effect of estrogen
   on postheparin lipolytic activity. J. of Clin. Invest.
   59, 601.
2. Beck, P. (1973): Contraceptive steroids. Modifications
   of carbohydrate and lipid metabolism. Metabolism 22,
   841.

3. Bennion, L.J., Ginsberg, R.L., Garnick, M.B., and Bennett, P.H. (1976): Effects of oral contraceptives on the gallbladder bile of normal women. New Eng. J. of Med. 294, 189.
4. Beral, V. (1976): Cardiovascular disease mortality trends and oral contraceptive use in young women. The Lancet 2, 1047.
5. Boyd, W.N., Burden, R.P. and Aber, G.M. (1975): Intra-renal vascular changes in patients receiving oestrogen containing compounds - a clinical histological and angiographic study. Quart. J. Med. (New Series XLIV), 175, 415.
6. Chait, A., Albers, J.J., Brunzell, J.D. and Hazzard, W.R. (1977: Type III Hyperlipoproteinaemia ('Remnant removal disease'). Insight into the pathogenetic mechanism. Lancet 1, 1176.
7. Hedlin, A.M. (1975): Effect of oral contraceptive estrogen on blood coagulation and fibrinolysis. Thromb. Diath. Haemorrh. 33, 370.
8. Hennekens, C.H. and MacMahon, B. (1977): Oral contraceptives and myocardial infarction. New Eng. J. of Med. 296, 1166.
9. Hollenberg, N.K., Williams, G.H., Burger, B., Chenitz, W., Hoosmand, I. and Adams, D.F. (1976): Renal blood flow and its response to angiotensin II: Interaction between oral contraceptive agents, sodium intake and the renin-angiotensin system in healthy young women. Circ. Res. 38, 35.
10. Katz, F.H. and Beck, P. (1974): Plasma renin activity, renin substrate and aldosterone during treatment with various oral contraceptives. J. Clin. Endocrinol. Metab. 39, 1001.

11. Mann, J.I., Inman, W.H.W. and Thorogood, M. (1975):
    Oral contraceptive use in older women and fatal myo-
    cardial infarction. British Med. J. 2, 445.

12. Martin, J.V., Martin, P.J. and Goldberg, D.M. (1976):
    Enzyme induction as a possible cause of increased serum
    triglycerides after oral contraceptives. The Lancet 1,
    1107.

13. Ory, H.W. (1977): Association between oral contracep-
    tives and myocardial infarction. J. Am. med. Ass. 237,
    2619.

14. Salhanick, H.A., Kipnis, D.M., and Wiele, R.L., van de
    (1969): Metabolic effects of gonadal hormones and con-
    traceptive steroids. Plenum Press. New York, London.

15. Terpstra, P. (1971): Orale contraceptiva, koolhydraat-
    stofwisseling en serum lipiden bij de mens. M.D. Thesis,
    Groningen.

CHAPTER VII

DEVELOPMENT OF HYPERTENSION

Birkenhäger, W.H., de Leeuw, P.W.,
Kho, T.L., Falke, H.E.

Patterns of blood pressure

Epidemiological studies on the incidence of primary
hypertension in Western countries have yielded frequencies
of 15 to 20 per cent. Obviously blood pressure is an erra-
tic variable; not only are there considerable intra-
individual variations during short-time observations, but
also age-related changes have been described. With increasing age the blood pressure tends to rise in Western
culture. Essential hypertension is characterized by a
steeper increase with age and a more marked involvement
of diastolic pressure.

The authors studied 207 essential hypertensives under
metabolic ward conditions. In this group the degree of
hypertension tended to be more severe in higher age groups,
even though the same criterium for the diagnosis of
hypertension was applied to all age groups. This feature
of a progressive disorder was not obvious during actual
follow-up studies. One explanation for this discrepancy
may be, that patients admitted to the follow-up study
were not under pressure to be treated effectively, because
generally there was no alarming progression. The blood
pressure profile was based on systematical in-patient
readings. When casual readings are taken into account, the

relationship with age should be less obvious, since blood pressure is accepted to be more labile in the young. We have assessed variability of blood pressure in a sample of patients, and found indeed a significant inverse relationship between variability of blood pressure and age. Even patients with hypertension starting at a higher age apparently do not disturb this general pattern. The regression is linear, there being no apparent distinction between patients with labile or more fixed hypertension. The incidence of labile hypertension differs in several studies, but for a great deal this seems to be due to problems of definition. Therefore, discussions on whether labile hypertension proceeds to sustained hypertension or not, mainly depend on presumptions. The natural history of labile hypertension has not been examined prospectively, although an excess risk of subsequent cardiovascular morbidity and mortality has been reported.

Cardiac output and calculated total peripheral vascular resistance

Blood pressure results from the interaction between cardiac output and total peripheral vascular resistance. Hypertension may be the result of an increase in either one of these factors or both. In the early days, it was generally thought that an increase in peripheral resistance was the main factor responsible for hypertension, although some authors stressed the importance of a high cardiac output. In later years this high output state has been recognized in a considerable number of patients, especially in those with only mild elevation of blood pressure. Although it is held by some authors that these patients form a special subgroup, the available data indicate a downward trend of cardiac output during the progression of the hypertensive disease. It is therefore possible that such patients represent an early stage of hypertension.

In most studies, the high cardiac output could be attributed to an increase in heart rate, stroke volume being normal. When excess cardiac function is mainly determined by heart rate, the underlying disorder has been attributed to a combination of sympathetic overactivity and parasympathetic inhibition. As a corollary it may be supposed, that these subjects at the time of the (invasive) measurements are more easily upset than their normotensive counterparts.

In our laboratory, all measurements are carried out after a sufficiently long time has passed for the patient to get accustomed to the environment. When our determinations of cardiac output in hypertensives are compared with those in normals (mainly adapted from the literature) a marked similarity is found. In fact, the relation between cardiac output and age in this study does not differ much from that in normals.

The decline in cardiac output with age is mainly caused by a reduction of stroke volume, which also occurs in normotensives.

The result of our cross-sectional study confirm the positive relationship of total peripheral vascular resistance and age. When the degree of hypertension is more severe, cardiac output seems to fall in the face of an increase in total peripheral resistance.

It can be inferred from these and other data that the natural history of hypertension is characterized by a steady increase in peripheral resistance.

However, when the haemodynamic studies from various laboratories are studied more closely, it appears that even at a stage when cardiac output is high, peripheral resistance is increased at the same time.

Renal haemodynamics and glomerular filtration

Although renal blood flow sometimes is normal in essential hypertension, in the majority of patients renal haemodynamics are abnormal. The general pattern is found to consist of a decrease in renal blood flow and an elevation of filtration fraction and renal vascular resistance. In our material we found evidence for a considerable impact of the hypertensive process on renal haemodynamics. The blood pressure level was inversely related to renal blood flow and glomerular filtration rate, and directly to filtration fraction. In the cross-sectional study we observed a negative relationship of renal blood flow with respect to age. As far as the duration of the hypertensive process is concerned, the longitudinal study showed a consistent and substantial decline with time.

In view of the physiological decrease in renal blood flow due to senescence, the progressive changes in the course of hypertension should be offset against the former. In normotensives no follow-up studies are available but the relationship between renal blood flow and age is well-documented. We have compared our results in the hypertensive patients with those reported for normal men and found that the reduction of R.B.F. (renal blood flow) with age for hypertensives is, generally, steeper than for normal subjects. The renal fraction is normal at an early stage of hypertension, but is progressively diminished. Changes in glomerular filtration rate become im-

portant only at a more advanced state, especially when
renal blood flow has fallen to values below 300 ml/min/m^2.

With a more refined technique (Xenon-washout) we
could demonstrate a significant decrease in outer cortical
blood flow already in early hypertension. This phenomenon
seems to be mainly responsible for the reduction of total
renal blood flow.

The findings with respect to renal haemodynamic
changes support the concept of an early increase in vascular resistance as the basic hypertensive mechanism.

The nature of the increase in resistance appears to
be complex. Both the functional and the structural components of the increase in renal vascular resistance can be
assessed by means of saline infusions or pharmacological
studies. Both components of the increase in resistance
may be the consequence of vasoconstrictor stimuli, either
originating from the tissues (auto-regulation) or from increased activity on the part of pressor systems.

A functional vasoconstriction has been thought to be
the result of auto-regulation of tissue blood flow in
response to an increased cardiac output. A main objection
to this view is that time relations do not fit the model.
Whereas a substantial increase in peripheral resistance
in essential hypertension takes many years, a firm auto-
regulatory control of tissue blood flow occurs much more
rapidly in experimental conditions where the ability of
the kidney to maintain extracellular fluid homeostasis is
tampered with.

Enhanced systemic pressor activity could be based
either on the renin-angiotension system or on the adrenergic system or both.

High renin levels are found in only a minority of patients with essential hypertension. This already casts some doubt on the assumption that increased activity of the renin-angiotensin system would play a role in the rise of vascular resistance. Moreover, in a number of patients plasma renin is abnormally low, a condition encountered in about one-third of the hypertensive population. In these cases renin is suppressed and unresponsive to stimuli as sodium restriction and tilting. The mechanism of the low renin state has not been elucidated thus far. Although several possibilities, including mineralocorticoid excess, volume expansion, electrolyte disturbances and reduction in sympathetic activity, have been proposed to characterize low renin hypertension as a distinct nosological entity, the evidence is far from conclusive.

Renin levels have been described to vary inversely with age in normotensives, although this is not a consistent finding. In hypertension such a relationship has been found more often.

In our cross-sectional study renin levels were also inversely related to age, at least up to 50 years. On the basis of these observations it can be postulated that the low renin state is a stage in the development of essential hypertension; in support of this idea is the negative relationship between renin and blood pressure observed in a number of studies. In our study renin was not clearly related to blood pressure, although there was an almost significant inverse relationship between these variables in the group with intact glomerular filtration rate. This suggests some feed-back suppression of renin at higher levels of blood pressure, as long as glomerular filtration is intact. Since these trends do not reach statistical significance, it is probable that blood pressure per se is not the only determinant of renin secretion.

We found that a rise in renal vascular resistance stimulates renin release. This was apparent for the cross-sectional as well as the follow-up study. Whether this is due to the accompanying reduction in glomerular filtration or to a greater fall in afferent arteriolar pressure, cannot be distinguished. It is unlikely that the rise in renal vascular resistance is caused by increased renin secretion, since these two parameters change in opposite directions in the early stages of hypertension.

It has been stated that aldosterone levels are lower in older (normotensive) age groups and at higher diastolic pressures. Since aldosterone secretion is dependent on several factors, including the renin-angiotensin system, most studies on this hormone have a dynamic, rather than a static character. In hypertensive subjects, the role of aldosterone production has mainly been investigated in the low-renin state. In these patients aldosterone secretion and excretion have been reported to be normal.

In our study plasma aldosterone was not related to age, blood pressure or P.R.C. It only showed a direct relation of borderline significance to extracellular (and interstitial) volume, but not to plasma volume.

It is unlikely therefore, that the renin-angiotensin-aldosterone system is of primary importance in the elaboration of essential hypertension.

As soon as substantial vascular alterations occur, the system apparently becomes geared into action, and may contribute to the development of malignant hypertension.

Pressor reactions could also be mediated via the alternative pathway, the adrenergic system. The activity of the adrenergic system is now being assessed by determining the level of circulating catecholamines, both in the steady state and during provocative manoevres.

There is still much controversy at this stage and a primary role of this system in the genesis of essential hypertension remains to be proven.

SUMMARY

This paper is based in part on a number of haemodynamic and endocrinological investigations in 207 patients with essential hypertension.

The general finding is an increase in total peripheral vascular resistance, which can be traced to an early stage of essential hypertension. In particular, this rise in resistance is found in the renal vasculature. The cause of the abnormal resistance remains unknown. Emphasis is given to the renin-angiotensin system, although in the final analysis this plays only a minor role. The adrenergic system is presently under scrutiny.

REFERENCES (overviews)

1) Birkenhäger, W.H. and Schalekamp, M.A.D.H. (1976): Control mechanisms in essential hypertension. Elsevier/North-Holland Biomedical Press, Amsterdam.
2) Borst, J.G.G. and Borst-de Geus A. (1963): Hypertension explained by Starling's theory of circulatory homeostasis. Lancet I, 677.
3) Brod, J. (1960): Essential hypertension: haemodynamic observations with a bearing on its pathogenesis. Lancet I, 773.

4) Dunn, M.J. and Tannan, R.L. (1974): Low-renin hypertension. Kidney Int. 5, 317.
5) Goldring, W. and Chasis, H. (1944): Hypertension and
   Hypertensive Disease. The Common Wealth Fund, New York.
6) Guyton, A.C. and Coleman, T.G. (1969): Quantitative
   analysis of the patho-physiology of hypertension. Circ.
   Res. 24 and 25, suppl. 1,1.

CHAPTER VIII
ENDOCRINE HYPERTENSION

Doorenbos, H.

Atherosclerosis is clinically evident in patients only when a vascular complication presents itself as the first unequivocal symptom of longstanding vascular disease. Hypertension may play a part in its causation, in turn it itself may develop on the basis of pre-existing atherosclerosis. Just as is the case with atherosclerosis, it is difficult to say where normal bloodpressure ends and hypertension begins. It is even more difficult to delinate endocrine hypertension as different from the mainstream of hypertension, being divided in low renin and high renin cases. Nevertheless the first clearly defined group of patients with low renin hypertension had endocrine disease nobody will dispute, i.e. primary aldosteronism. As it was soon found that many hypertensive patients belong to the low renin group, claims were made that primary aldosteronism is a very common disease, occurring in some 25% of all cases. The description of an entity called normokalemic hyperaldosteronism suggested that this might be so. Nevertheless present thinking allots only a small place to excess production of mineralocorticoids as a causative factor in low renin hypertension, even though claims have been made for overproduction of other salt-retaining steroids in this condition.

A better case can be made to call high renin hyper-

tension a form of endocrine hypertension. It is dependent
on a high level of angiotensin in the blood, a polypeptide
that not only makes the peripheral vessels contract, but
also induces increased secretion of adrenal aldosterone.
It has been shown to be active in the normal homeostatic
pressure mechanism, rising and falling in concentration
when effective blood volume is contracted or expanded. Administration of the angiotensin antagonist saralasin has
shown that under some circumstances even normal bloodpressure may be angiotensin dependent. This discussion will
not deal with renin angiotensin mechanisms as the subject
will be discussed elsewhere in the course. Endocrine dysfunction playing a minor or major role in the causation of
hypertension is seen in adrenal cortical hyperfunction, in
overproduction of catecholamines and in hyperparathyroidism.
It is also seen in those forms of adrenogenital syndrome
that have in common an overproduction of adrenal mineralocorticoids while cortisol secretion is diminished or almost absent. Hypertension caused by excess intake of succus
liquiritiae is partially due to a permissive action of endogenous cortisol. Hypertension in users of oral contraceptives is caused by a change in PRA equilibrium and will
not be discussed there.

Overproduction of cortisol is seen in the various
forms of *Cushing's syndrome*. It may be caused by an elevation of the hypothalamic/pituitary/cortisol feedbackset-
point,by ectopic production of ACTH and by autonomous hormone production in an adrenal adenoma or carcinoma. Cortisol
is a gluconeogenetic anti-inflammatory hormone with a salt-
retaining effect of such a degree, that it cannot be used
as a systemic corticoid when its antiphlogistic action is

desired. The early advent of synthetic cortisol analogues
has eliminated at least this undesirable effect of antiphlogistic therapy. In adult adrenalectomized patients a
daily dose of about 75 mg provides sufficient mineralocorticoid activity to maintain sodium balance. In most
cases of Cushing's syndrome cortisol production per 24
hours will be less than that, with the exception of cases
due to ectopic ACTH production and adrenal carcinoma.
Therefore the typical signs of mineralocorticoid excess i.e.
hypertension,   slight elevation of serum Na, slight fall
of serum K and a tendency to metabolic alkalosis in the
presence of renal potassium wasting,are usually not present.
It is to be expected, that low renin hypertension is present when there is retention of sodium. As atherosclerosis
makes its presence very much felt in Cushing's syndrome
that is pituitary dependent or caused by an adrenal adenoma
it is to be expected that vascular disease and hypertension
are prominent features. Cushing's syndrome is diagnosed
using low and high dexamethasone suppression tests.

Primary aldosteronism is a condition with overproduction
of the mineralocorticoid aldosterone usually in an adrenal
adenoma that results in mild hypertension with hypernatre-
mia, hypokalemia and metabolic alkalosis. Severe vascular
damage occurs only occasionally. The condition may be suspected in patients with aversion to salt, having polyuria
and polydipsia, muscle cramps and occasionally tetany. They
have a marked tendency to develop hypokalemia while using
small amounts of saluretics. Subjective and objective symptoms disappear when they are put on a salt restricted diet
or are given an aldosterone antagonist. Many cases will
remain undetected, because of the common practice to pre-

scribe salt restriction as first treatment of hypertension.
For differential diagnosis studies of PRA mechanism on a
high and a low salt regimen will have to be performed. High
renin malignant hypertension presents usually with a rather
different symptomatology; the distinction with "ordinary"
low renin hypertension may occasionally be difficult. The
rare syndrome of hyperreninism mimics primary aldosteronism.
It is doubtful whether aggressive diagnostic studies are
indicated to avoid overlooking probable primary aldosteronism as the clinical course is mostly mild, while the negative potassium balance can be corrected by giving potassium
sparing diuretic drugs. When potassium depletion is marked,
this results in metabolic alkalosis with tetany, in diminished renal concentrating ability, in diminished ability
to acidify the urine and to secrete hydrochloric acid in
the stomach, in diminished glucose tolerance due to impaired insulin secretion. Though extreme potassium deficiency has resulted in myocardial damage in animal experiments, there is no evidence of permanent cardiac damage
in man once the electrolyte abnormality has been corrected.
Also the disturbance of carbohydrate tolerance is rather
mild. Only few cases have been described of an adrenal carcinoma producing aldosterone in excess.

Congenital adrenal hyperplasia resulting in overproduction of salt-retaining adrenal steroids may induce hypertension. This is seen in 11- and in 17-hydroxylase deficiency. In *11-hydroxylase deficiency* the conversion of
compound S (11-desoxycortisol) in cortisol is impaired and
so is the conversion of desoxycorticosterone in corticosterone. The condition is diagnosed by the symptoms of early
accelerated growth with premature puberty in males and

82

virilization in females. Excretion of pregnanetriol, of desoxycorticosterone, of 11-desoxycortisol and of 11-desoxy-17-ketosteroids is increased. Plasma renin activity and aldosterone are suppressed. Treatment with cortisol suppresses the clinical and biochemical symptoms, the blood-pressure falls. It is not always possible to suppress ACTH production satisfactorily without risking some iatrogenic hypercorticism because of the height of the dose of gluco-corticoid needed. In *17-hydroxylase deficiency* the adrenal secretory ability of cortisol and the gonadal ability to secrete testosterone and estradiol are impaired, while des-oxycorticosterone, corticosterone and aldosterone are pro-duced in excess. This results in mineralocorticoid excess hypertension in individuals with   retarded growth, that do not go into puberty and have delayed skeletal matura-tion. Individuals with an XY chromosomal pattern may pre-sent themselves as phenotypic females. It is possible to suppress hypertension in these cases by administration of glucocorticoids. Replacement therapy with gonadal hormones has to be given in addition to induce and maintain secon-dary sexual characteristics.

The most frequently occurring type of endocrine hyper-tension is a catecholamine producing tumor, *a pheochromo-cytoma*. These tumors originate in the adrenal medulla or in sympathetic ganglia. In the adrenals they are bilateral in about 10% of cases. They secrete excess norepinephrin and epinephrin. The clinical picture consists of bouts of sweating, flushing or pallor with angina, palpitations and severe hypertension. There may also be a sustained eleva-tion of bloodpressure. Usually the symptoms are more im-pressive when the tumor is smaller, in large tumors the

catecholamines are already inactivated before they exert
a systemic effect. In patients presenting with medullary
carcinoma of the thyroid the presence of a pheochromocytoma
should always be suspected even when there is no clear cut
history of bouts of hypertension. The same is true for patients with neurofibromatosis. Diagnosis rests on the excretion of an excess of catechol metabolites as vanilyl-
mandelic acid and the metanephrines that both represent
about 40% of hormone production. When the metabolite excretion is not elevated provocation tests should be performed using preferentially glucagon and when no reaction
is seen also histamine. These tests are not without risk
and should never be performed without prior determination
of the excretion of catecholamines. Phentolamine should be
at hand, so that immediate measures can be taken, should a
positive reaction occur. When metabolic evidence has thus
been obtained suggesting a pheochromocytoma, after alpha
and beta blockade further röntgenologic studies should be
done to locate the tumor or tumors to be followed by surgical removal of the tumor.

Excess catecholamines hamper endogenous insulin secretion giving mild glucose intolerance. The PRA mechanism
may be stimulated because the bloodvolume is contracted
and by the action of catecholamines themselves. Thus a positive saralasin test may be found indicating that also in
this form of hypertension part of it may be angiotensin dependent. A hypertensive reaction due to the agonistpressor
action of saralasin has also been seen.

Hyperparathyroidism occasionally is diagnosed in a
patient with hypertension. It is well known, that administration of a thiazide diuretic potentiates parathormone

action and may induce hypercalcemia in susceptible individuals. When this persists following withdrawal of the medication a search is made for possible causes of hypercalcemia. After exclusion of other causes,if necessary using a
cortisone test according to Dent,a diagnosis of hyperparathyroidism is made. Determination of PTH may be of value
when used in conjunction with the serum calcium level. Successful surgery may or may not cure the hypertension. This
is not surprising, since in most cases of hyperparathyroidism renal damage caused by hypercalciuria is instrumental
in the origin and persistence of the high bloodpressure.
It is likely that the kidney plays a central role in the
hypertension of hyperparathyroidism, though there have been
some reports suggesting increased sensitivity of the vessel
wall to catecholamines in hypercalcemia.

Finally *gonadal dysgenesis* should be cited as a condition combining hypogonadism by chromosomal disturbance and
coarctation of the aorta and congenital kidney abnormality,
resulting in hypertension associated with but not caused by
endocrine disease. In typical cases diagnosis is not difficult, but many patients remain undiagnosed until puberty.
Weak or absent femoral pulses along with other stigmata of
the syndrome suggest the correct diagnosis of the hypertension.

Quantitatively endocrine hypertension is relatively
unimportant. A recent study from the Mayo clinic suggests
that its prevalence is even less then would be deduced from
publised series i.e. 0.18% of their patients underwent surgery for renal artery stenosis, 0.04% for pheochromocytoma
and 0.10% for aldosteronism, the respective numbers for the
frequency of Cushing's syndrome, hyperparathyroidism and

nonremediable endocrine pathology causing hypertension not being given. Yet it is important to recognize these rare cases in order to institute appropriate therapy.

Literature

1. Alvestrand, A., Bergström, J. and Wehle, B. (1977): Pheochromocytoma and renovascular hypertension. Acta Med. Scand. 202, 231.
2. Beevers, D.G., Brown, J.J., Ferris, J.B., Fraser, R., Lever, A.F. and Robertson, J.I.S. (1973): The use of spironolactone in the diagnosis and the treatment of hypertension associated with mineralocorticoid excess. Am. Heart J. 86, 404.
3. Bill, M. (1968): Neuroblastoma, newer chemical diagnostic tests. JAMA 205, 103.
4. Buchem, F.S.P. van, Doorenbos, H. and Elings, H.S. (1956): Primary aldosteronism due to adrenocortical hyperplasia. Lancet 2, 335.
5. Conn, J.W., (1955): Primary aldosteronism, a new clinical syndrome. J. Lab. Clin. Med. 45, 3.
6. Conn, J.W. (1965): Hypertension, the potassium ion and impaired carbohydrate tolerance. New Engl. J. Med. 273, 1135.
7. Conn, J.W., Rovner, D.R. and Nesbit, R. (1966): Normokalemic primary aldosteronism. JAMA 195, 21.
8. Conn, J.W., Rovner, D.R. and Cohen, E.L. (1968): Liquorice induced pseudoaldosteronism. JAMA 205, 492.
9. Christy, N.P. and Laragh, J.H. (1961): Pathogenesis of hypokalemic alkalosis in Cushing's syndrome. New Engl. J. Med. 265, 1083.

10. Doorenbos, H., Cost, W.S. and Nagelsmit, W.F. (1960): The effect of aldosterone antagonists on disturbance of carbohydrate metabolism in primary aldosteronism. Acta Endocr. Kbh. Suppl., 185.

11. Dunn, F.G., Carvalho, J.G.R. de, Kern, D.C., Higgins, J.R. and Fröhlich, E.D. (1976): Pheochromocytoma crisis induced by saralasin. New Engl. J. Med. 295, 605.

12. Earl, J.E., Kurtzman, N.A. and Moser, R.H. (1966): Hypercalcemia and hypertension. Ann. Int. Med. 64, 378.

13. Editorial (1976): Solving the adrenal lesion of primary aldosteronism. New Engl. J. Med. 204, 441.

14. Hoogdalen, P. van, Donker, A.J.M., Brentjens, J.R.H., Hem, G.K. van der and Oosterhuis, J.W. (1977): Partial correction of hypertension by angiotensin II blockade in a patient with pheochromocytoma. Acta Med. Scand. 201, 395.

15. Krakoff, L.R., Nicolis, G. and Amsel, B. (1975): Pathogenesis of hypertension in Cushing's syndrome. Am. J. Med. 58, 216.

16. Kaplan, M.M. (1969): Commentary on incidence of primary aldosteronism. Arch. Int. Med. 123, 152.

17. Lange, W.E. de, Lappöhn, R.E., Sluiter, W.J. and Doorenbos, H. (1977): Primäre Amenorrhoe und Hypokaliämie infolge 17 alpha hydroxylase Mangels. Deutsche Med. Wchnschr. 102, 1024.

18. Lange, W.E. de, Weeke, A., Artz, W., Jansen, W. and Doorenbos, H. (1973): Primary amenorrhea with hypertension due to 17 hydroxylase deficiency. Acta Med. Scand. 193, 565.

19. Lawrence, A.M. (1967): Glucagon provocative test for phaeochromocytoma. Ann. Int. Med. 66, 1091.

20. Plaen, J.F. de, Boemer, F. and Yperseele de Strihou, C. van (1976): Hypercalcaemic phaeochromocytoma. B.M.J. 2, 734.

21. Roth, G.M. and Kvale, W.F. (1945): A sensitive test for phaeochromocytoma. Am. J. Med. Sc. 210, 653.

22. Tucker, R.M. and Labarthe, D.R. (1977): Frequency of surgical treatment for hypertension in adults at the Mayo Clinic from 1973 through 1975. Mayo Clinic Proc. 53, 549.

CHAPTER IX
RENAL FUNCTION AND ATHEROSCLEROSIS

Birkenhäger, W.H., Kho, T.L., de Leeuw, P.W.,
Wester, A.

It is difficult to dissociate the effects of disturbances of kidney function on degenerative vascular disease, from those brought about by hypertension. Atherosclerosis is a disorder in which high blood pressure according to epidemiological findings is one of the main aetio-
logical factors. There is also evidence that the localized
nature and topographical distribution of atheroma result
from the action of haemodynamic alterations. The mechanical stress caused by altered pressure and flow may well be
a major determinant in the siting of atheromatous plaques.
Pressure is possibly more important in the early stage,
while the finishing touch to the development of a plaque
is determined more by (local) metabolic or homeostatic
aberrations.

In experimental pathology interest has mostly been
focussed on the genesis of *arteriolar* lesions in severe
hypertension. It is commonly held that such lesions are
probably the direct mechanical result of raised arterial
pressure, whatever the cause. Nevertheless, it has been
suggested that some product of the kidney contributes
directly to vascular damage, by exerting a "vasculotoxic"
effect. Goldblatt[6] supposed that a high pressure might act
together with a toxic substance of renal origin to produce

arteriolar lesions. The substance responsible for the vascular damage is of course recognizable as angiotensin II.

The role of altered renal function can be analyzed by establishing different forms of hypertension and studying the incidence of early arteriolar damage. Such early lesions can be traced by submitting rats to carbon injections at a comparable level of pressure, e.g. 180-200 mmHg systolic. When different aetiologies of experimental hypertension (DOCA-salt, renal artery constriction, angiotensin infusion) are compared in this respect, the focal lesions are similar. In all groups the same degree of endothelial damage with granular material and colloidal carbon particles displacing the media smooth muscle is observed[7,8].

Observations in animals with so-called renoprival hypertension have shown that not even the presence of the kidney is a necessary condition for the introduction of hypertensive arteriolar necrosis. In view of these results the renin-angiotensin system is not implicated in the development of vascular damage. Nevertheless the concept has been developed by Laragh and his coworkers that renin or its products have a direct vasculotoxic effect that could contribute to the occurrence of strokes and myocardial infarct[1,2]. Fifty nine of 219 hypertensive patients had low plasma renin levels and did not develop strokes or heart attacks, in contrast to the other patients (with normal or high levels) who exhibited an 11-14 % incidence of these complications. The suggestion that renin adds to the risk of hypertension per se has been widely accepted, even though it actually has received less support[3] than opposition[4,5,9,10]. To many workers the concept that the development of arteriolar lesions and atheroma in larger

arteries would be based on the same mechanism was difficult to accept.

In 1968 we started a prospective investigation to
record changes with time in patients with uncomplicated
essential hypertension. Sixty-three white patients (after
a treatment pause of at least 14 days) were studied under
metabolic ward conditions. During the in-hospital sodium
intake was 60 milli-equivalents per day. The intake was
checked by determination of 24 hours sodium excretion.
Thus, optimal conditions were obtained for distinguishing
an abnormally low renin level from normal and high levels,
according to the criteria proposed later by Brunner et al.
[1,2].

Blood samples for the measurement of plasma renin con-
concentration were taken between 09.00 and 10.00 hours,
after the patient had been recumbent for at least one
hour. Plasma renin concentration was determined according
to the method described by Skinner[11], followed by bio-
assay and/or radioimmunoassay[12]. Arterial pressure was
measured intra-arterially in the recumbent patient between
10.00 and 12.00 hours, using a Statham transducer. Calcu-
lation of renal blood flow was based on measurements of
$0-(^{125}I)$-iodohippurate-clearance from 10.00 to 12.00 hours.
Renal extraction of $0-(^{125}I)$-iodohippurate was either
determined directly or it was assumed to be 74 %, this
being the average value established in our laboratory.

Patients remained under surveillance in the out-
patient department. They were treated with varying combinations of propranolol, methyldopa and clonidine. The drugs
were not selected according to renin levels. Patients were
definitely undertreated by their own volition (because of
side-effects). Almost without exception a diastolic blood

pressure between 95 and 115 mm Hg was obtained in the sitting position. The average period of surveillance was 54 months.

Patients in whom complications occurred were readmitted into our department. Those who met with myocardial infarction were restudied after clinical recovery.

Results

In this population of patients with uncomplicated hypertension at the time of the first examination elevated plasma renin levels were exceptional. By contrast, low renin hypertension was frequently observed.

Cardiovascular complications were observed in 11 patients, after an average period of 29 months (3-48 months). Seven patients were proven to have myocardial infarction and four met with a stroke.

The distribution of initial renin levels in the 11 patients with complications covered nearly the entire "hypertensive range", but a slight prevalence of low-renin hypertension was observed. The patients were divided into two subgroups (low renin and normal/high renin).

Table 1 shows the clinical characteristics in the two groups. The low renin patients on the average were somewhat older than those with normal or high renin levels, and the average blood pressure in the first group was lower. The differences were not significant. There was no difference in other risk factors (overweight, diabetes, smoking and serum cholesterol).
Renal vascular resistance was used as a parameter of vascular constriction. The resistance values in the 11 patients in whom complications occurred were distributed in an even spread across the entire range.

TABLE 1 - Clinical characteristics of patients with cardiovascular complications

Renin Subgroup	Number (Males)		Age[*]	Mean[*] Blood Pressure	Plasma Renin Concentration
			Years	mm HG	ng ml^{-1}h^{-1}
Low	6	(4)	56	137 ± 10[+]	2.7 ± 0.3
Normal/High	5	(3)	50	147 ± 21	10.7 ± 5.5

[*] No significant differences between subgroups

[+] Mean ± SD

In 6 patients with myocardial infarction plasma renin concentration was determined after clinical recovery. On the average a significant rise was observed in comparison with the initial values. Thus the results of this prospective study fail to confirm the claim, that a medium or high plasma renin level can be implicated as an added risk factor with respect to the incidence of heart attack and stroke [1,2]. We were also unable to substantiate the notion, that low-renin hypertension represents a less vasoconstricted state than hypertension with higher renin levels[13]. In addition, our findings indicate that a high renal vascular resistance, which indicates small-vessel involvement, has little in common with large-vessel complications. Finally, our results indicate that a rise in renin is one of the sequelae of myocardial infarction, rather than being a contributary factor. This fact could explain -at least in part- the difference between our findings and the results of the original retrospective study[1,2].

It seems to be highly unlikely, therefore, that alterations in renal function, otherwise than by raising blood pressure, contribute to the genesis of atherosclerosis. This should be considered to be a preliminary conclusion, since future clinical investigations may quite well reveal the finding, that such functions as prostaglandine-synthesis by the kidney will be reflected in varying patterns of atherosclerosis.

REFERENCES

1. Brunner, H.R., Laragh, J.H. and Baer, L. et al. (1972): Essential hypertension: renin and aldosterone, heart attack and stroke. N. Engl. J. Med. 286, 441.
2. Brunner, H.R., Sealy, J.E. and Laragh, J.H. (1973): Renin as a risk factor in essential hypertension: more evidence. Am. J. Med. 55, 295.
3. Christlieb, A.R., Gleason, R.E and Hickler, R.B. et al. (1974): Renin: a risk factor for cardiovascular disease? Ann. Intern. Med. 81, 7.
4. Doyle, A.E., Jerums, G. and Johnston, C.I. et al. (1973): Plasma renin levels and vascular complications in hypertension. Br. Med. J. 2, 206.
5. Genest, J., Boucher, R. and Kuchel, O. et al. (1973): Renin in hypertension: how important as a risk factor? Can. Med. Assoc. J. 109, 475.
6. Goldblatt, H. (1938): Studies on experimental hypertension. J. Exp. Med. 67, 809.

7. Goldby, F.S. (1975): The vascular pathology of hypertension. In: Hypertension - its nature and treatment,
   p. 55. Ed. D.M. Burley, G.F.B. Birdwood, J.H. Fryer,
   S.H. Taylor. CIBA, Horsham, England.

8. Goldby, F.S. (1976): The arteriolar lesions of steroid
   hypertension in rats. Clin. Sci. Molec. Med. 51, 315.

9. Mroczek, W.J., Finnerty, F.A. and Catt, K.J. (1973):
   Lack of association between plasma-renin and history
   of heart attack or stroke in patients with essential
   hypertension. Lancet 2, 464.

10. Stroobandt, R., Fagard, R. and Amery, A. (1973): Are
    patients with essential hypertension and low renin
    protected against stroke and heart attack? Am. Heart J.
    86, 781.

11. Skinner, S.L. (1967): Improved assay methods for renin
    "concentration" and "activity" in human plasma. Circ.
    Res. 20, 391.

12. Schalekamp, M.A.D.H., Schalekamp-Kuyken, M.P.A. and
    De Moor-Fruytier, M. et al. (1973): Interrelations
    between blood pressure, renin, renin substrate and
    blood volume in terminal renal failure. Clin. Sci.
    Molec. Med. 45, 417.

13. Laragh, J.H. (1973): Hypertension manual, p. 823. Ed.
    J.H. Laragh, Dun-Donnelly Corp. New York.

CHAPTER X
CARDIAC MANIFESTATIONS OF ATHEROSCLEROSIS

Nieveen, J., Groningen, The Netherlands

INTRODUCTION

The three most important cardiac manifestations of atherosclerosis are:
1. stable angina pectoris
2. unstable angina pectoris (impending infarction)
3. myocardial infarction

The symptomatology, diagnostic procedures and current treatment will be discussed in this paper with the exception of the treatment of myocardial infarction, which will be described in the paper of Arntzenius: "Modern therapy of myocardial infarction" (chapter XII).

Stable angina pectoris

This disease is caused by a discongruence between need and supply of coronary arterial blood during exercise, emotional stress or changing of environmental temperature.

Diagnostic procedures

A. History

The history of these patients is very important for the diagnosis. For reasons of standardisation it is wise to use the questionnaire of the World Health Organisation, designed by the London School of Hygiene and Tropical Medicine (Rose and Blackburn, 1968). This questionnaire distinguishes between two grades of angina pectoris: type 1 is the light form with the following criteria: chest complaints do exist, occuring during walking uphill or hurrying on the level, but not during walking at an ordinary pace on the level; one stops or slows down or carries on after taking a tablet of nitroglycerin under the tongue, the feeling hereby disappears and it does so in 10 minutes or more quickly, the feeling is located retrosternally and/ or in the left anterior chest, but in the latter case in the left arm also. Type 2 is the severe form in which the questions are answered like in type 1, but with the addition of complaints during walking at an ordinary pace on the level.

Increasingly more frequent the so-called "variant" angina pectoris (Prinzmetal) is described in the literature.

In these cases chest complaints occur during the night with patients lying in bed without exertion. It is probably that mostly spasms of coronary arteries are the cause of the complaints, in contradiction to the usual angina pectoris, where complaints develop during exertion, which causes imbalance of the coronary circulation due to atherosclerotic narrowing of the coronary arteries.

B. Exercise electrocardiography

In most patients with angina pectoris the resting ECG is normal. Many tests have been developed in the last decades in order to study the electrocardiogram during exercise. The oldest method was the two-step-test described by Master (1935).

More sophisticated tests have been developed since. Ascoop (1974) described in his thesis the diagnostic value of various criteria of exercise electro- and vectorcardiography and also the significance of some of these criteria in predicting the anatomical localisation of coronary artery obstructions was evaluated. He used a graded exercise test at the same time recording the electrocardiogram, which was analysed with the aid of a computer. After recording the ECG at rest, the patients sitting on a bicycle-ergometer, were loaded with 30 Watts. Every 3 minutes the load was increased by 30 Watts until one of the following stop-criteria was reached:

A. Occurrence of angina pectoris
B. Manifestation of ischaemic ST depression with a junction depression of more than 2 mm
C. The appearance of conduction disturbances (atrioventricular or intraventricular)
D. Appearance of repetitive ventricular extrasystoles, totalling more than 8 % of the total number of complexes per minute
E. Complaints of tiredness, dizzines etc.

After stopping the exercise during the recovery phase every minute for 7 minutes an ECG is recorded. During the test it was attempted to reach a workload, which produced a heartrate of at least 90 % of the age corrected predicted maximum heartrate. These normal standard values have been determined by Sheffield et al. (1965) in normal subjects of different age classes during exercise tests, in which normal O_2 uptake was also determined. The results of these exercise tests were correlated with the anatomical findings of the coronary arteries during coronary arteriography (Ascoop, 1974) and are shown in Table 1.

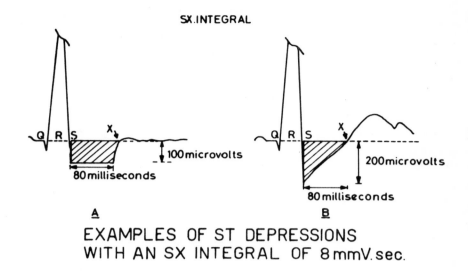

SX.INTEGRAL

**EXAMPLES OF ST DEPRESSIONS
WITH AN SX INTEGRAL OF 8 mmV.sec.**

Fig. 1. Measuring of the SX integral (from Ascoop 1974).

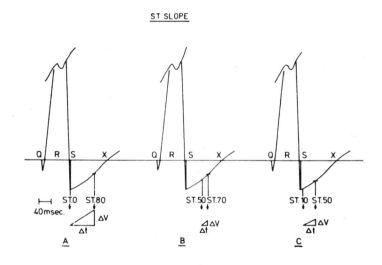

ST SLOPE

Fig. 2. Measurements of the ST slope using different intervals (from Ascoop 1974).

TABLE 1 - Comparison of the diagnostic value of various criteria for one single lead. Result of exercise test related to findings of coronary arteriography in 87 patients

Criterion	Leads	Correct positive fraction	Correct negative fraction	Index of Merit
Ischaemic ST segment (XECG)	CM5	0.17*	1.00	0.17 ($\pm$ 0.10)
SX integral	CC5	0.39	1.00	0.39 ($\pm$ 0.09)
ST slope $\triangle V/\triangle t$ (0-80)	X	0.61	0.90	0.51 ($\pm$ 0.09)
ST slope [$\triangle V/\triangle t$(50-70), ST(50)]	X	0.68	0.90	0.58 ($\pm$ 0.08)
ST slope [$\triangle V/\triangle t$(10-50), ST(10)]	CC5	0.72	0.90	0.62 ($\pm$ 0.08)

* This low sensitivity is partly explained by the basis on which the patients are selected

An ischaemic ST depression is defined as follows:
a. if during exercise there appears a junction depression of at least 100 mV with regard to the baseline
b. and if this junction depression is followed by horizontal sagging of the ST segment of at least 80 msec duration

The ST integral is the amplitude time integral beneath the iso-electric line (Fig. 1). The measurement of the ST slope at different time points is shown in Fig. 2. As is shown in Table 1, the best correlation between exercise test and coronary angiogram was found with the ST slope between 10 and 50 msec combined with the amplitude of the ST depression at point 10 msec after S. However, there is not a 100 % correlation, but the results of the ischaemic

ST segment measurements are poor. Using more leads (14)
according to Chaitman et al. (1977) seems to improve still
more the sensitivity and efficiency of the maximal exercise test.

In Groningen and Utrecht (Antonius Hospital) the ST
integral and ST slope between 10 and 15 msec combined with
the amplitude of the ST depression at point 10 msec after
the S point during exercise are used as criteria for
ischaemic heart disease.

Fig. 3 shows 2 examples of the trend of the ST integral during exercise in a patient with significant coronary obstruction (CAG pos) and in a normal subject (CAG
neg.) and Fig. 4 the results of comparing the ST slope
(10-50 msec) and ST depression at point 10 msec with the
findings at coronary angiography in 87 patients (Ascoop,
1974). A quite good separation of positive and negative
coronary angiograms is found. These results can be obtained
most easily with the help of a computer, but it should
also be possible to measure these things by hand.

C. An other newer diagnostic procedure is the combination
of exercise and the use of radio-active substances as
Thallium ^{201} (^{201}Tl.) (Zaret, 1977).

After intravenous injection of radio-active Thallium^{201}
this substance accumulates in the cells of the heart-
muscle. In regions with decreased coronary circulation the
uptake is less than in normal parts of the heart. It is
possible to measure the radio-activity in the heart exter-
nally with the help of a scintillation camera. The procedure, which is used in the departments of Cardiology and
Isotopes in Groningen (Van den Berg, Woldring et al.) is
as follows:

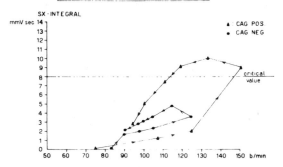

Fig. 3. The course of the ST integral during exercise in a patient with significant coronary obstructions (CAG pos.) and in a normal subject (CAG neg.) (from Ascoop 1974).

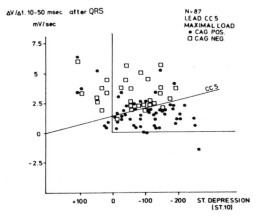

Fig. 4. Relation between ST slope and ST depression [ΔV/Δt (10-50), ST (10)], in dependence on the findings at coronary arteriography (from Ascoop 1974).

The patient is exercised on an ergometer as described above. At the moment he complains of chestpain or ST depressions occur in the ECG: 2 mcu Thallium[201] is injected intravenously. The exercise is continued for another minu-

102

te to allow adequate distribution of the tracer. 10-15 minutes later imaging is started and pictures are made of the myocardium in anterior - 45° left anterior oblique - and transverse positions. One hour later restscans are made in the same positions and the pictures are compared to the post-exercise pictures.

Fig. 5 shows schematically the distribution of the coronary arteries over the myocardium and the spread of the radio-active substance in the different regions (. . . . . = radio-activity).

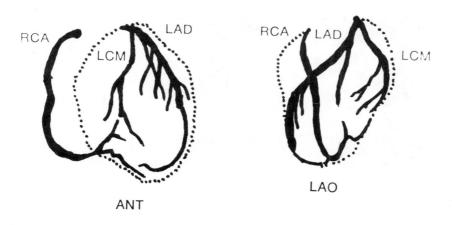

Fig. 5. See text

Fig. 6 shows a) a restscan, b) a post-exercise scan and c) a post-operative scan of a patient with angina pectoris. Already in the resting phase, but more during exercise, there is diminished radio-activity in the inferior-anterior part of the left ventricle. After coronary artery operation (c) there is a good spread of radio-activity over

a

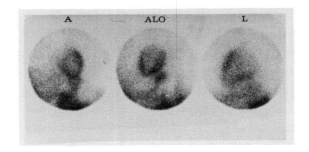

b

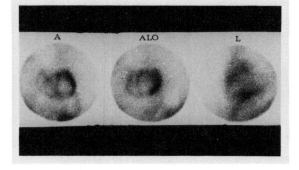

c

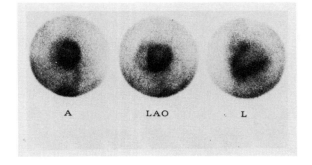

Fig. 6 a, b, c. See text

the heart. Van den Berg in our clinic compared the results of these examinations with coronary angiography and found a good correlation.

It is not possible to determine the exact narrowing of the coronary arteries with this method, only ischaemic regions can be detected. For localisation of stops or narrowings in the coronary arteries one has to perform selective coronary arteriography.

D. Selective coronary arteriography

Special preformed catheters can be positioned in the coronary arteries via a brachial artery (Sones, 1962, 1974) or via Seldinger needles in a femoral artery (Judkins, 1968). Contrast medium such as urografin 76 % is injected manually and cinefilms are made of the contrast-filled coronary arteries in different positions. So the exact places and spread of atherosclerosis of the coronary arteries can be visualised. Fig. 7 shows an example of a narrowing in the left anterior descending coronary artery.

Treatment of angina pectoris

In the first place it is necessary to take general measures, such as treating overweight (less calories, more physical activity and so on), lipid metabolism disturbances (cholesterol-, triglycerides-lowering diets), stop smoking, treating hypertension and diabetes. The drugs of choice are now:
1. stopping an attack of angina pectoris or prevent an attack the patient knowing certain forms of exertion provoking attacks: nitroglycerin sublingualy ½-1 mgr. This drug produces a decrease in arterial pressure,

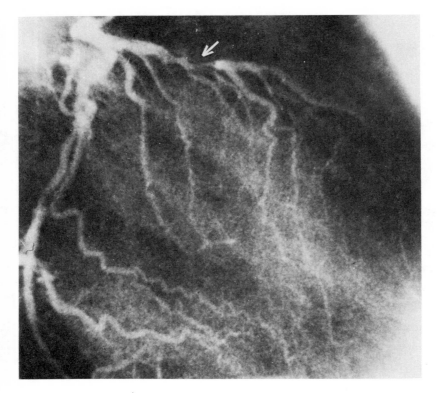

= narrowing LAD branch

Fig. 7. See text

veno-dilatation with decreased venous return, possibly
some vasodilatation of still reactable coronary arteries.
2. prophylactic treatment with beta-adrenergic blocking
agents, such as propranolol, alprenolol, metoprolol,
oxprenolol, pindolol a.s.o. These drugs cause: decrease
of myocardial contractility, - pulse rate - bloodpressure - stroke output a.s.o., so reducing the oxygen
consumption of the myocardium.

3. Eventually also long-acting nitrates as isosorbide-
dinitrate, 4 dd 5 mgr can be added. The effect of these
drugs lasts 2 to 3 hours.

In patients not reacting sufficiently on this conservative treatment, surgical treatment should be considered.
The possibilities of surgical treatment depend on the de-
fects found at coronary angiography. The surgeon uses in
operable cases pieces of the saphenous vein to bypass
stops and narrowings of coronary arteries. With this
operation the atherosclerotic process is of course not
cured, but in many patients the anginal pains disappear.

The life expectancy of patients treated surgically
or medically seems to be equal according to recent literature (Braunwald, 1977). Murphy et al. (1977) reported the
results of 596 patients with stable angina, randomized
into a medical group (310 patients) and a surgical group
(286 patients). Patients with left-main coronary artery
disease were excluded. The operative mortality at 30 days
was 5.6 %. Approximately one year after operation 69 % of
all grafts were patent and 88 % of the surgical patients
had at least one patent graft. There was no statistically
significant difference in survival at a minimal follow-up
interval of 21 months between patients treated medically
and those treated surgically. At 36 months 87 % of the
medical group and 88 % of the surgical group were alive.
However, the complaints of angina pectoris were distinctly
lower in the surgical than in the medical group. An exception is made for patients with narrowing of the main branch
of the left coronary artery. In these cases surgical treatment has proven to lengthen life and these patients should
have operation early (Takaro et al., 1976).

Unstable angina pectoris (impending infarction)

This can be:
1. increasing attacks of angina pectoris, suddenly starting first only during exercise, later also during resting
2. increasing angina pectoris after a long symptomfree period following myocardial infarction
3. more frequent and longer lasting attacks of angina pectoris without good reaction on nitroglycerin in patients with stable angina pectoris during months or years

The diagnosis should be made mainly by good history-taking. During attackfree periods the ECG is mostly normal, but during pain ECG-abnormalities (ST depression, T wave changes a.s.o.) occur. There are two ways of treatment for this syndrome: a) The more conservative consists of bedrest, anticoagulants and beta-receptor-blockers as described above; b) A more aggressive approach is the acute coronary angiography followed (if possible) by coronary surgery. In the literature there is not yet agreement which method should be preferred. There is some accordance about mortality: equal in both medical and surgical treatment groups. The medical patients having more angina than the surgically treated patients. Scheidt (1977) reported the results of a randomized trial with 288 patients having unstable angina, treated medically or surgically. In the hospital phase mortality was comparable in both groups (medical 4.1 %, surgical 5 %). Also in the post-hospital phase, averaging 24 months mortality was equal (medical 5 %, surgical 5.2 %). The surgically treated patients had a higher incidence of myocardial infarction (18 %) in the hospital than the medically treated group (10 %), whereas in the 24 months post-hospital phase the incidence was equal in both groups (13 %).

Myocardial infarction

The third manifestation of atherosclerosis of the coronary arteries is myocardial infarction. Mostly sudden occlusion of an atherosclerotic narrowed coronary artery causes long-lasting ischaemia of a part of the heart-muscle. The chest complaints are the same as described with angina pectoris, but stronger, lasting longer, start-ing suddenly and not especially occuring during exercise. The patients are mostly very ill, vomit, the blood pres-sure goes down and most frequently cardiac arrythmias occur. The most dangerous arrythmia is ventricular fi-brillation, leading to death, unless immediately cardiac resuscitation (heart massage, artificial breathing) and electrical defibrillation is started. The patients have to be sent as soon as possible to a coronary care unit in a hospital in order to control the heartrythm and to defi-brillate in case of ventricular arrythmias, such as ven-tricular fibrillation. The modern treatment of myocardial infarction and the problem of sudden death will be discus-sed in the papers of Arntzenius and Dunning (chapters XII and XI).

Diagnosis of myocardial infarction

As in angina pectoris history is important (see above). In most cases the diagnosis can be confirmed by the electrocardiogram or vectorcardiogram. The three typical signs in the ECG in myocardial infarction are ST-elevation (caused by the zone of injury at the border of the infarction), T-wave changes (caused by ischaemia around the infarction) and deep QS-waves (caused by des-truction of cardiac muscle).

With the different leads of the ECG or the vector-cardiogram, it is possible to localize the infarction: anterior, inferior, posterior, anteroseptal or combinations of these. Not in all cases the ECG is abnormal in the beginning. In these cases it is important that we have *laboratory* methods to conclude to myocardial damage. The most sensitive enzyme to appear in the circulation after destruction of cardiac muscle is creatinephosphokinase (C.P.K.).

The measurement of C.P.K. has proven to be a useful tool in the diagnosis of myocardial infarction (Sobel, 1972). In cases of concomitant skeletal muscle damage an elevated total C.P.K. adds, however, little information, because of the C.P.K. originating from the skeletal muscle. The quantification of the so-called M.B. iso-enzyme, which is found almost exclusively in heart muscle, provided a more specific indication of myocardial infarction than total C.P.K. alone. Initially the quantification techniques were too laborious and time-consuming for most clinical laboratories.

Varat and Mercer (1975) described an ion-exchange chromatographic technique more simple than older methods. Roche Diagnostics (1976) developed therefore the C.P.K.-C.S. (Roche T.M.) cardiac specific C.P.K. iso-enzyme system, a highly specific and sensitive diagnostic indicator, which is readily available to most hospital laboratories. Varat et al. expressed the C.P.K.-M.B. as a percentage of the simultaneously determined total serum C.P.K. They examined 100 consecutive admissions to the coronary care unit. In 47 patients with proven myocardial infarction, including 3 with normal total C.P.K. the peak M.B. was greater than 4 % of total C.P.K. In 49 patients

without infarction, including 15 with elevated total C.P.K.
(due to trauma, injections, cardioversion), the peak M.B.
was less than 2 % of total C.P.K. The M.B. band was elevated, but did not peak in 4 patients without infarction,
but with chronic atrial fibrillation. So the determination
and quantification of C.P.K.-M.B. iso-enzyme and expressing
it in percentage of total C.P.K. is a very important new
diagnostic in patients with possible myocardial infarction,
when the ECG is still normal, in patients with small infarctions and to detect recurrences of myocardial infarction during the observation of the patient.

With serial determinations of the C.P.K.-M.B. concentration in the blood, it is also possible to get an impression of the size of the infarction and to observe the
results of treatment with certain drugs (for instance beta-
receptor blocking agents).

Other enzymes, somewhat later occuring than C.P.K.,
are the serum-glutamic-oxaloacetic-transaminase (SGOT)
and still later the lacto-dehydrogenase (LHD). The larger
the infarction, the higher and long-lasting the levels of
enzymes.

Of course, also elevation of leucocytes, blood sedi-
mentation rate and temperature is caused by the destruction of cardiac muscle. The above described radio-nuclear
method with Thallium^{201} is also applicable in myocardial
infarction patients in order to determine the size of the
infarction. This method, however, is not yet generally
used.

Besides arrythmias other complications of myocardial
infarction are: cardiogenic shock, cardiac failure, rupture of the intraventricular septum and of the papillary
muscles of the mitral valve causing mitral insufficiency,

rupture of the myocardium causing tamponade of the heart, aneurysms of the heart muscle at the site of the infarction and systemic arterial emboli.

In the Western World the increase of patients with angina pectoris and myocardial infarction at younger ages (30-50 years), in the last 25 years is of epidemic size, probably caused by the modern living habits in these parts of the world. We have to treat as good as possible all patients with angina pectoris and myocardial infarction, but still more important is to advocate strongly: prevention of coronary heart disease by changing these modern living habits, or try in other countries not to take over these wrong habits of the Western World.

LITERATURE

1. Ascoop, C.A. (1974): ST forces during exercise, Academic Thesis, Groningen.
2. Braunwald, E. (1977): Coronary artery surgery at the crossroads. New England Journal, 297, 661.
3. Chaitman, B.R., Wagniart, C., Corbara, F., Bourassa, M.G. (1977): Improving the efficiency of the graded exercise test. Circulation, 56-III-7, 1977.
4. Judkins, M.P. (1968): Percutaneous transfemoral selective coronary arteriography. Radiologic Clinics of North America, VI, 467.
5. Master, A.M. (1935): The two-step-test of myocardual function. American Heart Journal, 10, 4, 95.
6. Murphy, M.L., Hultgren, H.N., Detre, K., Thomsen, P.H.J., Takaro, T. (1977): Treatment of chronic stable angina: a preliminary report of survival data of the randomized Veterans Administration Coop. Study. New England Journal of Medicine, 297, 621.

7. Roche Diagnostics (1976): Cardiac enzymes in perspective. Roche 340, Kingsland Street, Nutley, New Jersey, 07110.

8. Rose, G.A., Blackburn, H. (1968): Cardio-vascular survey methods. W.H.O. monograph, no. 56. World Health Organisation, Geneva.

9. Scheidt, S. (1977): Unstable angina: medical management of surgery. Cardiovasc. Med., 2, 541.

10. Sheffield, L.T., Holt, J.H., Reeves, T.J. (1965): Exercise graded by heartrate in electrocardiographic testing for angina pectoris. Circulation, 32, 622.

11. Sobel, B.E., Shell, W.E. (1972): Serum enzyme determinations in the diagnosis and assessment of myocardial infarction. Circulation, 45, 471.

12. Sones, F.M., Shirey, E.K. (1962): Cinecoronary arteriography. Modern Conc. Cardiovascular Dis., 31, 735.

13. Sones, F.M. (1974): Coronary cinearteriography, in Willis Hurst, The Heart P. 377. McGraw-Hill book company.

14. Takaro, T., Hultgren, H.N., Lipton, M.J. (1976): The V.A. cooperative randomized study of surgery for coronary arterial occlusive disease. II Subgroup with significant left main lesions. Circulation, 54, suppl. 3-III, 107-III 117.

15. Varat, M.A., Mercer, D.W. (1975): Cardiac specific creatinephosphokinase iso-enzyme in the diagnosis of acute myocardial infarction. Circulation, 51, 855.

16. Zaret, B.L. (1977): Myocardial imaging with radioactive potassium and its analogs. Progress in cardiovascular diseases, 20, 81.

Acknowledgment: The author is grateful to Dr. C.A. Ascoop for the permission to use some of the figures of his thesis.

CHAPTER XI
SUDDEN CARDIAC DEATH: SOME CLINICAL ASPECTS

Dunning, A.J.

Sudden, unexpected death is a difficult subject for analysis. It occurs mostly outside the hospital or shortly after arriving, without medical attendance or even unwitnessed. Its magnitude, importance and threat in contemporary Western societies, however, is such that it should be defined, studied and hopefully prevented. Major attention will be given to the latter, but a rational approach is only possible when the setting and mechanism of sudden cardiac death is known.

Frequency of sudden cardiac death

It is generally assumed and sometimes proven that the majority of sudden, unexpected and non-violent deaths is cardiac by nature and mostly caused by severe coronary artery disease. These data are derived from reports of coroners or medical examiners in major cities or as an endpoint in assessing its prevalence in a group of already identified patients, e.g. after myocardial infarction.

Since medicolegal practice differs between states and cities and only autopsy can establish a more or less certain diagnosis, these reports must show a definite bias.

Generally it appears that in the middle age, between

40 and 70 years, about a quarter of all certified deaths are sudden. When only autopsied cases are analysed, it appears that even in older reports cardiac death accounts for at least half the deaths.

When sudden death is defined as occurring within one hour after the onset of the acute episode and this episode being witnessed, an incidence of coronary heart disease in men was 91%, in women 52% in a study done in New York in the fifties.

In two cities, Rochester in Minnesota and Malmö in Sweden, sudden death was studied in the community where sudden death both outside and in the hospital was reviewed. Coronary artery disease was the leading cause. Sudden death may be a manifestation or even late result from clinically overt coronary heart disease as well as its initial manifestation. In all prospective studies on sudden death in previously healthy individuals, coronary heart disease is the cause in 20 to 25 percent. Thus, sudden death may occur in healthy people as well as in survivors of coronary events and risk assessment for any individual is therefore extremely difficult.

It appears likely, that sudden cardiac death occurs more frequently at a younger age, ten times more in men, especially in blacks. From the Baltimore study on sudden death and myocardial infarction it appeared that white men had a higher incidence of transmural infarction and more coronary thrombi when sudden death occurred, while black men had more ventricular hypertrophy. Women smoked more, were frequently unmarried and, unexpectedly, had more psychiatric problems in their history. The setting of sudden death is highly variable, but strenuous physical activity is unusual. Stress, whether physical or mental, preceded sudden death in no more than a quarter of all males and only a minority of females in the Stockholm study.

Predisposing factors in sudden cardiac death

Sudden death is often thought to be the result of acute myocardial infarction at the beginning of the ischemic period and it seems likely that risk factors for coronary heart disease predispose in the same manner for sudden cardiac death. Thus, in an American study in Pittsburgh, a severe form of coronary artery disease with at least three vessel disease with 75% narrowing was found at autopsy in the majority of males, many of them having old myocardial infarctions. Single artery disease was uncommon and only a third of all persons dying suddenly had no prior history of heart disease or medical care. In the patients, who died both suddenly and unexpectedly in apparently good health, always major obstructions in multiple coronary arteries was seen.

Although the background of sudden cardiac death usually is severe coronary artery narrowing, an acute myocardial infarction due to a recent coronary thrombosis is often not present. These thrombi may form a secondary phenomenon after the event and their prevalence is dependent on survival time. Thus, thrombotic occlusion leading to infarction and ventricular fibrillation in most autopsy studies had the low frequency of only 20 to 30 percent.

When a coronary profile was related to the occurrence of sudden death in prospective studies like those in

Framingham and Albany, the risk of sudden death could be estimated from these well-known risk factors. One third of sudden deaths occurred in men in the upper ten percent of risk profiles but increasing age, previous clinical manifestations of coronary heart disease or a specific combination of risk factors could not identify those at maximal risk. Thus, the risk results, demonstrating themselves in a changed coronary artery anatomy and blood flow, have more influence than risk factors on clinical manifestation, a critical proximal obstruction being the most significant.

Therefore given a certain degree of silent or manifest coronary artery obstruction, death may occur in relation to electrophysiologic disturbances rather than sudden and new occlusions.

Identification of high risks of sudden death

Since evidence from mobile and hospital coronary care units have demonstrated ventricular fibrillation as the most likely cause of sudden cardiac death, the risk of this arrhythmia is important to assess. For years it has been presumed that premature ventricular beats were harbingers of ventricular fibrillation, especially in the early phase of acute myocardial infarction. The premature beats have been considered warning arrhythmias, the suppression of which, especially by lidocaine, was indicated.

In recent years, however, it has become evident that ventricular fibrillation may strike out of the blue without any warning, whereas premature ventricular beats in the ischemic heart may or may not lead to ventricular fibrillation. This implies that prevention of ventricular

fibrillation should be extended to all patients in the
early phase of myocardial infarction, irrespective of the
presence of ventricular premature beats.

The question arises whether all premature ventricular
beats are equal or some are more equal than others. The
answer is dependent on the time and duration of cardiac
monitoring: one must consider that a 12 lead electrocardiogram barely represents one minute of monitoring. A
human heart beats a 100.000 times a day and it requires
sophisticated data compression and processing to determine
the incidence and type of ventricular premature beats.

When patients with clinical coronary heart disease,
whether sustained infarction or angina pectoris, are
monitored during 24 hours, about 85 percent of them show
ventricular premature beats. In 17 percent this will be
occasional, in 25 percent multiform and in 30 percent repetitive, and the severity is greater after myocardial
infarction than in angina pectoris. When compared to the
extent and grade of coronary artery obstruction during
angiography, the severity of the ventricular arrhythmias
is clearly related to the extent of the disease.

Instead of 24-hour monitoring maximal exercise tests
may reveal severe ventricular arrhythmias in the same
patients, although it is less effective. Sympathetic
activity may be the link between ventricular irritability
and stress, since during sleep the grade and quantity of
premature beats is minimal while maximal during exercise
in multivessel disease.

Even shorter periods of monitoring may identify high
risk patients. In a recent study over 1700 men with prior
myocardial infarction were monitored for ectopic activity

for only one hour and following during two years. When complex premature beats occurred (R on T, runs of ectopics, multiform premature beats, bigeminy) in the monitoring hour, the likelihood of sudden death increased threefold against men without such arrhythmias.

Thus, a coronary risk profile, the presence of clinical coronary heart disease and the occurrence of complex premature ventricular beats, either during long-term monitoring or provoked by exercise, may more or less define the candidate for sudden death. However, the outline of that portrait is rather vague when it comes to selecting candidates for prevention.

Approaches towards prevention of sudden cardiac death

Current approaches towards the prevention of sudden cardiac death can be thought of as four concentric circles with increasing radius, the outer one trying to prevent the basic disease process, coronary artery disease in the community, the innermost one trying to save an individual from imminent cardiac death; the other two circles include pharmacotherapeutic measures either at danger points or prophylactically after survival of a coronary event. In the city of Seattle a comprehensive, rapid response emergency system has been in operation since 1970. The fire department, coupled to coronary care units, provides easy patient access and is trained for cardiopulmonary resuscitation. Apart from that the public has been alerted and trained and about 80.000 citizens of Seattle, a one and a half million city spread over 200 square kilometers, have been trained in resuscitation techniques. This means that nearly one in five resuscitation procedures is started

by persons on the scene before the rescue squad arrives.
Thus in five years 1106 patients were treated for ventricular fibrillation outside the hospital, from which 234
survived and were discharged home after hospitalization.
Only 10% of these patients had evidence of an acute myocardial infarction and in at least 55% data were adequate
to rule out tissue necrosis. The most disquieting fact in
this study was the poor prognosis of patients who survived
ventricular fibrillation without infarction, their mortality being three times higher than in fibrillation
occurring with infarction. The acute ventricular excit-
ability during infarction may be temporary, but recurrence
may be common if there is chronic instability without
muscle necrosis.

As far as historical information was present, ventricular fibrillation was the first manifestation of coronary heart disease in a third of those patients, while a
positive history of coronary heart disease could be ascertained in nearly half of this group. Coronary arteriography
in a small subgroup of survivors demonstrated rather severe
obstruction in the majority.

When the balance is made, in Seattle about 40% of all
victims of ventricular fibrillation are now resuscitated
and one out of four leaves hospital. Prognosis, however,
is exceptionally poor when there is no underlying infarction, a frequent finding confirmed by others. Recurrence of ventricular fibrillation in the next six months
is likely and prodromal symptoms are usually absent,
making some form of preventive pharmacotherapy highly de-
sirable.

A second approach is to identify the candidate for

sudden death, e.g. those patients surviving their first myocardial infarction or those having angina pectoris. These patients are included in a surveillance system in which they communicate with a local coronary care unit by telephone transmission. With a simple electronic device they can transmit their electrocardiogram by telephone in case of chest pain, arrhythmia or other warning signals. Before enrolling in this system they are given auto-injectors with lidocaine and atropine and trained to use them when directed. Since the danger of ventricular fibrillation or severe bradycardia is the greatest just after the onset of symptoms, the patient can protect himself during at least one hour by injecting either lidocaine or atropine intramuscularly, before a cardiac ambulance reaches him and transport to hospital is effected. The system requires a high-grade technology, a well-trained and motivated patient, but provides pharmacological intervention at the earliest moment of ischemia caused by myocardial infarction.

A recent approach to prevention of sudden cardiac death by drug therapy has been tried in Sweden and England. In both trials a beta-blocking drug, either practolol or alprenolol, was given to patients surviving their first myocardial infarction.

In the Swedish study, concerning 230 patients, the control group after two years showed 11 cardiac deaths against 3 in the treated group. In the British multicentre study 3000 patients were followed in 67 hospitals, but the side-effects of practolol, then beginning to emerge, resulted in an untimely end. Again, in the treated group of 1500 patients 30 sudden cardiac deaths occurred against 52 in the placebo-group. Further analysis showed that patients with low body weight - and probably relatively high practolol plasmalevels - and a past anterior infarction benefitted most. It has to be remembered that for every survivor nearly 75 patients have to be treated, exposing them to side-effects of unknown severity.

The latest trial reported in this setting was done in the U.S. with the drug Anturane (sulfinpyrazone), formerly used for gout and known to inhibit platelet adhesion and aggregation in vitro. In a group of 1475 patients surviving a first myocardial infarction a double-blind study was done and follow-up was only 8.4 months, the most critical period after infarction as to the risk of sudden death. The difference between treated and placebo-group was surprising, since the annual sudden cardiac death rate was 6.3 percent in the placebo-group against 2.7 percent in the treated group. When these data hold true, the sudden cardiac death rate in the first year after infarction can be halved, thus saving the lives of some 20.000 Americans annually.

Caution, however, is necessary, since sudden cardiac death is only partially a sequel to a coronary event while patient compliance and side-effects may limit the usefulness of long-term preventive drug therapy.

Those engaged in preventive cardiology, at the outer perimeter of our specialty, urge a more fundamental approach. Althought the benefit/risk ratio of any drug therapy may be acceptable or even favourable, the burden of premature coronary death warrants wider measures. These are only partly medical, since our life style has become a risk factor and any modification of it requires the acceptance of the community. In a follow-up study in

Chicago, consisting of 900 middle-aged men free of disease in 1958, none of them died suddenly in the next 10 years and only three in the next 15 years. Those of the same group having a diastolic blood pressure over 90 mm Hg, a cholesterol over 250 mg/L or smoking more than 10 cigarettes a day, had a long-term mortality three times that of the others. Public taste changes and fat and food consumption is gradually altering, while more effective measures are instituted to detect and treat hypertension. Cigarette smoking, especially in the young, however, is increasing in nearly every country, whatever the government undertakes to curb the habit.

Thus, the paradox of our health scheme is to spend money on coronary care units, cardiac ambulances and cardiac surgery, all of them coping with the end points of coronary heart disease through costly and sophisticated technology. On the other hand, because of a life style promoted by affluence and advertising, we are unable to stem the tide that inevitably washes us to the shore of coronary heart disease and its ultimate expression, cardiac death.

Literature

1. Sudden coronary death outside hospital. Circulation (1975): 52, Suppl. III.
2. Improvement in prognosis of myocardial infarction by longterm beta-adrenoreceptor blockade using practolol. Brit. Med. J. (1975): 2, 735.
3. Wilhelmsson, C. et al. (1974): Reduction of sudden deaths after myocardial infarction by treatment with alprenolol. Lancet 2, 1157.

4. Sulfinpyrazone in the prevention of cardiac death after
   myocardial infarction. New Engl. J. Med. (1978): 298,
   289.
5. Fehmers, M.C.O. and Dunning, A.J. (1972): Intramuscularly and orally administered lidocaine in the treatment of ventricular arrhythmias in acute myocardial
   infarction. Am. J. Cardiol. 29, 514.

CHAPTER XII
MODERN THERAPY OF ACUTE MYOCARDIAL INFARCTION

Arntzenius, A.C. and Oudhof, J.H.

1. The use of the Coronary Care Unit (CCU)
2. Bedrest, ambulation, duration of hospital stay
3. General treatment of patients with acute myocardial infarction
4. Arrhythmias and their treatment
5. Treatment of heart failure and cardiogenic shock
6. Coronary angiography in the acute stage of myocardial infarction

1. THE USE OF THE CORONARY CARE UNIT (CCU)

The Coronary Care Unit has generally been accepted as the required surrounding to monitor patients with acute myocardial infarction (AMI). In particular arrhythmias (to which these patients are prone) can be detected and treated at an early stage. The hospital mortality of AMI as a result, has dropped from 25-30 % in the pre-CCU period to around 15 % at present (Table 1). Recently in some CCU's, not only is the cardiac rhythm monitored, but also the systemic blood pressure and occasionally the pulmonary artery pressure or the "wedge" pressure. With trend changes in these hemodynamic signs heart failure and cardiogenic shock can be diagnosed and treated more effectively.

TABLE 1 - Hospital mortality in acute myocardial infarction and age (CCU, Leiden).

Age (years)	<40	40-49	50-59	60-69	70-79	> 80
Percentage dead during hospitaliz-ation for A.M.I.	0	7	14	15	17	23

As myocardial infarct patients are generally quite understandably upset and often in a distraught state, care should be taken in the CCU, to combat the psychological trauma of the onset of the disease. The CCU should there-fore be as quiet as possible and certainly not located nextdoor to the intensive care, as is occasionally seen.

The patient, as soon as admitted, should be given an explanation preferably by the nurse or the physician about his or her situation, and the diagnosis and the equipment used. A mild sedative and a sleeping medication are usually prescribed. It is our habit to provide patient with an in-travenous drip and to monitor the ECG signal right away. Needless to say that physician and nurses should work har-moniously together to create the required environment of quietness, confidence and understanding.

2. BEDREST, AMBULATION, DURATION OF HOSPITAL STAY

No longer do we prescribe six weeks bedrest. Manage-ment has been liberalized since the early fifties. Mobili-zation on the fourteenth day has been shown to be no less satisfactory than prolonged regimens of bedrest for uncom-plicated cases and is now common practice in most CCU's. Others have mobilized patients with uncomplicated infarctions as early as the eighth day.

It should be stressed however, that patients with heartfailure, persistent pain, recurrent arrhythmias, cardiomegaly or evidence of aneurysm obviously require longer periods of rest.

Once the patient is allowed to get up, a regimen should be provided for, by which the patient is gradually allowed to use more of his muscles each day.

In Leiden patients with presumably small myocardial infarctions with CPK values of less than 250 without serious arrhythmias and in whom the pain has subsided within 24 hours, mobilization begins on the second day and is completed after 10-14 days. With AMI's which produce CPK values of between 250 and 900 and with arrhythmias, mobilization depends on the disappearance of arrhythmias. The scheme is slower and will be completed between 14 and 21 days. There is no rule or limit to be given for AMI patients who develop heartfailure, cardiogenic shock, the mobilization can take as long as 4 weeks or even longer.

3. GENERAL TREATMENT OF PATIENTS WITH AMI

Complete bedrest during the first two to seven days after which patient is allowed to walk to the bathroom with help. An intravenous route is opened up immediately after admission to CCU. This provides for an easy way to administer drugs as a bolus when urgently required.

Oxygen supplementation by nasal prongs (2 l/min or more as required) is advised in most instances, because patients with AMI are usually hypoxemic.

Relief of pain

In the first few hours often dilaudid[R] (morphia) or demerol[R] (pethidine) is required for initial control of the pain of MI. We routinely use thalamonal[R] (droperidol and fentanyl combined) 1-2 ml with slow push intravenously. With persisting and serious pains it is our habit to administer vilan[R] (a morphine derivate).

It is not unusual for patients with acute MI to have residual chest pain for 2-3 days after the acute event. The pain may also be caused by pericarditis and auscultation should help to diagnose the latter condition.

All anginal episodes should be promptly treated with sublingal nitroglycerine or cedocard[R] (isosorbide-dinitrate).

Anticoagulants

Deep vein thrombosis is not uncommon in patients with acute MI. We would therefore like to recommend to use anticoagulant treatment routinely in patients with acute myocardial infarctions unless a definite contra-indication is found to be present. Anticoagulant therapy in acute myocardial infarction prevents venous thrombosis, pulmonary embolism and mural thrombus formation. In particular anticoagulant treatment is indicated in patients with congestive heart failure, low-output syndrome or patients confined to bed for a prolonged period of time. Anticoagulants are contra-indicated when there is pericardial effusion since they may precipitate bleeding into the pericardial space. Generally as soon as the pericardial effusion is over, anticoagulant treatment in AMI can be reinstated. Anticoagulants should also be withheld in patients with hemorrhagic complications and in those with very high blood pressures.

The diet

In the first 24 hours after onset of AMI, usually a liquid diet is given. Next a so-called "soft" diet is prescribed. We routinely restrict sodium intake to help prevent cardiac failure and lower blood pressure. Generally a fat restricted, low cholesterol and caloric reduced diet is prescribed.

4. ARRHYTHMIAS AND THEIR TREATMENT

Sinus bradycardia

To be treated only when accompanied by low blood pressure or ventricular premature beats (VPB's): atropin 0.5-1.0 mg.

Sinus tachycardia

- If the underlying cause is heart failure, it should be treated with intravenous furosemide and digoxin intravenous.
- If there is hypovolemia, plasma or dextran or glucose 5 % may be required.
  Sedate and relief pain when required; also look for infection and for pericarditis.

Atrial fibrillation

When ventricular rate is rapid try cardioversion or administer intravenous digoxin[R]: 0.25 mg every 4 hours.

Atrial flutter

Very often the heart rate will be 150 and a 2:1 AV conduction ratio exists. Cardioversion is the treatment of choice.

Atrial premature beats (APB's)

Atrial premature beats are common in AMI and generally do not require treatment. They may result from congestive heart failure, hypoxia or electrolyte disturbance which should be diagnosed and treated.

Junctional rhythms

Slow junctional (nodal) rhythm is usually an escape mechanism and often does not require treatment as long as ventricular rate is adequate. If however, this gets slow (less than 40/min) and there appear ventricular premature beats, then an artificial pacemaker is indicated, after first atropine is tried.

Rapid junctional rhythms may have their origin in digitalis overdosage and carotid massage and cardioversion should be considered like in cases of paroxysmal atrial tachycardia.

Ventricular premature beats (VPB's)

Very frequently seen in patients with AMI. Potentially dangerous are:
- A VPB frequency greater than 5/min
- Multifocal VPB's
- R on T phenomenon (R falls on T wave of preceding beat)
- Ventricular bigeminy
- Couplets (pairs) of VPB's

VPB's can be due to ischemia, anxiety, hypokalemia and Congestive Heart Failure, and these conditions should be diagnosed and whenever possible be corrected.

Lidocaine administered intravenously is the most widely used agent for the treatment of ventricular irritability. Give 50-100 mg bolus of lidocaine I.V. followed by infusion of 2-4 mg/min. Later the infusion rate can be lowered to 1 mg/min. If however, ventricular ectopy still is not suppressed add procainamide 500 mg. I.V. by slow push (5 min) followed by infusion of 4-6 gr/24 hours.

Quinidinesulphate may be given orally 200-400 mg every 6 hours for chronic suppression of ventricular ectopy or else try rythmodan[R] (disopyramide) 4-6 times 100 mg per day.

Ventricular fibrillation

Immediate cardioversion with 300 or 400 watt/sec is essential. If reversion of spontaneous rhythm does not occur, closed chest cardiac massage, endotracheal intubation and intravenous bicarbonate should be given, followed by renewed attempts of cardioversion after injection of bolus of 100 mg of lidocain I.V. When spontaneous rhythm occurs intravenous lidocain should be given for at least 24 hours.

Indication for artificial pacemaker

Complete Heart Block with a slow ventricular rate or Adams-Stokes attacks is an indication for pacemaker insertion. Patients who develop Mobitz type II conduction disturbance, if associated with an anterior M.I. or fascicular block deserve to get a temporary pacemaker inserted.

Pacing is usually not indicated with Wenckebach phenomena. A new RBBB during anterior infarction should be considered for insertion of a temporary pacemaker.

Slow junctional rates should be paced and so should all slow rhythms if low blood pressure develops not responding to repeat doses of atropine.

It is our practice in Leiden as regards insertion of artificial pacemakers in patients with AMI to generally withhold the treatment when the infarction is located inferiorly, but on the other hand not to hesitate with this type of therapy in patients with infarction of the anterior wall.

5. TREATMENT OF HEART FAILURE AND CARDIOGENIC SHOCK

Treatment of congestive heart failure

Bedrest promotes diuresis and should be given. Sodium restriction is mandatory. Prophylactic anticoagulants is indicated to reduce the risk of pulmonary emboli. Diuretics: lasix[R] (furosemide) with potassium replacement or potassium sparing diuretics such as dytac[R] (triamtereen) or moduretic[R] (amiloride and hydrochlorothiazide).

Treatment of Left Ventricular Failure

In pulmonary edema morphinesulphate gives beneficial relief in anxiety, decrease in tachypneu and decline in peripheral vascular resistance. Rotating tourniquets and phlebotomy may be helpful.

Oxygen is indicated and so are a rapidly acting intravenously given diuretic (furosemide) and intravenous digoxin[R] or ouabain[R]. If tachycardia or signs of left ventricular failure persist despite digoxin and repeated furosemide injections, nitroprusside should be considered, when the blood pressure is 110 mmHg or more and nitroglycerine can be used even with lower blood pressures.

Occasionally patients with severe persistent left ventricular failure can be stabilized with intra-aortic balloon counter pulsation.

Cardiogenic shock

Patients with acute myocardial infarction with a systemic blood pressure of less than 90 mmHg (2x measured) or with blood pressure far below their usual blood pressure and having an urine output less than 20-30 ml/hr are thought to be in shock. Their skin is cool, clammy and they have a depressed mental state. These patients should be monitored for cardiac rhythm, systemic blood pressure and pulmonary artery and"wedge"pressure. If the"wedge" pressure is less than 10 mmHg, the patient probably is hypovolemic and rapidly he (or she) should be infused with 5% glucose solutions or haemaccel. If on the other hand the"wedge"pressure is elevated (20 mmHg or above) treatment as described under left ventricular failure should be instituted and intra-aortic balloon pumping be considered. In Leiden we use *intra-aortic balloon pumping* in cardiogenic shock with persisting crushing pain ($\geqslant$ 24 hrs) when combined with S-T segment elevations and when there are recurrent ventricular tachy-arrhythmias, refractory to drug treatment. Occasionally also the Prinzmetal syndrome or patients with main stem lesions of the left coronary artery can be treated with this type of cardiac assist device. It is also used in patients with poor LV function just prior to or after surgical intervention.

By using the intra aortic balloon pump the systolic
arterial pressure and thus the afterload is lowered and
the diastolic coronary artery filling pressure is elevated, promoting coronary blood flow that way.

6. CORONARY ANGIOGRAPHY IN THE ACUTE STAGE OF MYOCARDIAL INFARCTION

In our coronary care unit at Leiden it has in the
past few years become customary to investigate a group of
complicated cases of acute myocardial infarction (in up
to 22 %) with coronary angiography. This group includes
patients with refractory cardiogenic shock, with recurrent
ventricular tachycardia fibrillation or patients with
persisting unstable angina. In the latter case first β-
blockade and nitrates are given. But when they do not
result in improvement, visualization of the coronaries is
indicated, and surgery is considered. Surgical intervention
for such patients usually consists of a coronary bypass
with occasionally infarctectomy or aneurysmectomy.

Mortality depends to a high degree on the residual
function of the left ventricle: if this is little the mortality is high.

Recently Ezra Amsterdam et al. have concluded from
results observed in their centre that it is important and
feasible to identify by means of left heart catheterization and angiography, those patients with cardiogenic shock
or recurrent ventricular tachycardio-fibrillation intrac-
table to conventional medical therapy who have surgically
approachable lesions. They state that in patients thus
selected for emergency surgical therapy, approximately
60 per cent achieve long-term survival following cardiac
operation. Since about one-half of patients with refrac-

tory pump failure due to AMI are appropriate candidates for angiographic evalutation of which group, potentially correctable lesions by operation are found in two-thirds of the individuals, it follows that ultimately in approximately 20 per cent of AMI patients with cardiogenic shock chronic survival can be expected to occur.

SUGGESTED READING

1. Alpert, J.S., Francis, G.S. Manual for Coronary Care. Little, Brown and Company, Boston, 1977.
2. Amsterdam, E.A. et al. Acute myocardial infarction shock: Operative intervention and results. Advances in heart disease, v.I. Edited by Dean T. Mason. Grune & Stratton.
3. Sobel, B.E. The cardiac care unit, 1974. In: E. Braunwald, ed. The Myocardium: Failure and Infarction, New York: HP Publishing Co., Inc., 1974.
4. Killip, T., Kimball, J.T. Treatment of myocardial infarction in a coronary care unit. Am. J. Cardiol., 20, 457, 1967.
5. Peel, A.A.F., Semple, T. Immediate prognosis in acute myocardial infarction. In: L.E. Meltzer and A.J. Dunning eds., Text book of Coronary Care. Philadelphia: The Charles Press, 1972.
6. Swan, H.J.C., Blackburn, H.W., DeSanctis, R., Frommer, P.L., Hurst, J.W., Paul, O., Wallace, A., Weinberg, S. Duration of hospitalization in "uncomplicated completed acute myocardial infarction". Am. J. Cardiol., 37, 413, 1976.
7. Maroko, P.R., Radvany, P., Braunwald, E., Hale, S.L. Reduction of infarct size by oxygen inhalation following

acute coronary occlusion. Circulation, 52, 360, 1975.

8. Schamroth, L. How to approach an arrhythmia. Circulation, 47, 420, 1973.

9. Chatterjee, K., Swan, H.J.C. Vasodilator therapy in acute myocardial infarction. Mod. Concepts Cardiovasc. Dis., 43, 119, 1974.

10. Favaloro, R.G., Effler, D.B., Cheanvechai, C., Quint, R.A., Sones, F.M. Jr. Acute coronary insufficiency (impending myocardial infarction and myocardial infarction) - surgical treatment by the saphenous vein graft technique. Am. J. Cardiol., 28, 598, 1971.

11. Swan, H.J.C., Ganz, W., Forrester, J., Marcus, H., Diamond, G., Chomette, D. Catheterization of the heart in man with the use of flow-directed balloon-tipped catheter. N. Engl. J. Med., 283, 447, 1970.

CHAPTER XIII
HYPERTRIGLYCERIDEMIA IN DIABETES MELLITUS

Sailer, S.

A clinical observation, the frequent coexistence of endogenous hypertriglyceridemia and carbohydrate intolerance, suggests that these two symptoms are related to each other or even influence each other. Since hypertriglyceridemia and diabetes mellitus are well-known risk factors for the development of atherosclerosis, the relationship between diabetes and hypertriglyceridemia is of very high clinical significance. Further, the understanding of the pathophysiological mechanisms of this interrelationship should form the basis of a successful treatment of these risk factors.

1. Hypertriglyceridemia in juvenile onset diabetes with insulin deficiency.

This type of hypertriglyceridemia was observed very frequently in patients with juvenile onset diabetes in the pre-insulin era treated with a fat rich diet. The milky plasma was called "diabetic lipemia". It was shown that in these severely diabetic patients with ketoacidosis mainly the chylomicron fraction is grossly elevated with low levels of LDL and normal HDL concentrations. On the contrary, a normal lipoprotein concentration and distribution have been observed in juvenile diabetic patients that were under good control with insulin.

In careful studies it was shown that patients with uncontrolled juvenile diabetes and ketoacidosis have massive hypertriglyceridemia on a 40% fat diet with plasma triglycerides as high as 7500 mg%, but on a 0% fat diet triglyceride levels returned to normal levels within a few days. The post-heparin lipolytic activity was subnormal.

From *in vitro* studies we know that insulin is required for the synthesis of lipoprotein lipase respectively for maintaining normal lipoprotein lipase activity and adequate triglyceride removal. This explains the fact that especially a fat rich diet leads to gross hypertriglyceridemia in insulin deficient patients.

Thus, this form of diabetic hypertriglyceridemia can be classified as a form of fat-induced lipemia secundary to chronic insulin deficiency as seen in some forms of juvenile diabetes. Not only diet control but also appropriate insulin therapy is effective in clearing the hypertriglyceridemia.

2. *Hypertriglyceridemia in maturity onset diabetes.*

In the plasma of this type of diabetes mellitus a normal or increased concentration of insulin, a moderate elevation of glucose, an increased concentration of free fatty acids, and an increased concentration of triglycerides are found. Mainly the very low density lipoprotein fraction is elevated. Activity of lipoprotein lipase and the removal of plasma triglycerides are normal. Since in these patients an elevated glucose concentration in the plasma does not (to the same extense as in normals) suppress the liberation of free fatty acids from adipose tissue adequately, the uptake of free fatty acids by the liver is increased as a result of their high plasma concentration; the fraction of free fatty acids taken up by the liver, which is esterified to triglycerides and secreted into the blood stream as very low density lipoprotein-triglyceride is high. Thus, an increased flux of "endogenous" plasma triglycerides from the liver into the blood occurs in this situation and is responsible for the hypertriglyceridemia.

It could be shown quite clearly, that only by an excellent control of diabetes (mainly by dietetic regimens, avoiding any overweight) the increased concentration of triglycerides can be reduced.

3. *Decreased glucose tolerance in patients with endogenous hypertriglyceridemia.*

Most cases of endogenous hypertriglyceridemia are accompanied by mildly impaired glucose tolerance, which is caused not by an insulin deficiency, but by an insuline resistance. This phenomenon is not confined to a certain "lipoprotein pattern" of hyperlipoproteinemia. Today we do not understand the pathomechanism of this insulin resistance completely. Some pathogenic mechanisms have been put forward to explain the common association of insulin resistance with endogenous hypertriglyceridemia:
1) It may simply reflect the common occurrence of obesity in hypertriglyceridemic persons.
2) Alterations in triglyceride metabolism resulting from hypertriglyceridemia per se may impede the action of insulin.

3) Insensitivity to insulin may be an intrinsic component of at least some primary hypertriglyceridemic states.
4) An alteration in insulin receptors may be in part resonsible for insulin resistance, at least in obese patients.

The fact has to be stressed, however, that in most patients with primary endogenous hypertriglyceridemia, hyperinsulinemia, insulin resistance, decreased glucose tolerance, and obesity, the administration of insulin does not lead to a lowered plasma triglyceride concentration, but, probably due to increased caloric intake after insulin administration, to an increase in body weight and in triglyceride concentration.

Actually, we do also not know at this moment whether hyperinsulinemia combined with hyperglucosemia leads to hypertriglyceridemia, but many factors speak against such a hypothesis.

As far as therapeutic measures concern, a dramatic improvement of the metabolic situation (decrease of plasma triglycerides and glucose) can be achieved by an hypocaloric diet.

CHAPTER XIV
GLUCOSE REGULATION AND THE DEVELOPMENT OF MICRO-
ANGIOPATHY IN DIABETES MELLITUS

Reitsma, W.D.

The relation between metabolic control of diabetes
mellitus and the risk of the occurrence of late complications, especially diabetic microangiopathy has been an open
question for many years. The presence of microangiopathy in
patients with mild maturity onset diabetes mellitus and the
lack of signs of microangiopathy in some patients with a
juvenile type of diabetes mellitus have been used as an
argument against the relation between metabolic control and
microangiopathy. This trend of thought was supported by Siperstein e.a., who claimed the occurrence of thickening of
the muscular capillary basal membrane in genetic diabetics
before glucose intolerance develops (Siperstein e.a. 1968).
They also did not find a relationship between basal membrane thickness and the duration of hyperglycemia. On the
other hand Kilo et al. did not find a thickening of the
muscular basal membrane before the occurrence of glucose
intolerance.(Kilo e.a. 1972). Other authors could not even
demonstrate a thickening of the basal membrane of muscular
capillaries in patients with juvenile diabetes of recent
onset. (Danowski e.a. 1972, Jordan and Perley 1972). The
significance of muscular capillary basal membrane thickening has been a matter of dispute in the literature for
several years. Recently the literature on fixation techniques,
methods and the obtained results has been reviewed. (William-

son and Kilo 1977). One of the conclusions is, that it is
now definitely established, that an increased thickness of
the muscular capillary basal membrane does not occur in
diabetes mellitus before the development of glucose intolerance.

Diabetic microangiopathy of the retinal, glomerular,
muscle and skin capillaries is characterized by a thickening of the basal membrane and a proliferation of the endothelial cells. Functional alterations like a labile microcirculation with changing dilatation of the small arteries,
the small veins and the capillaries precede and accompany
small vessel lesions and contribute to the development of
more advanced degenerative microangiopathy. There is also
an increase of capillary flow and plasma permeability.
These early functional changes are probably due to fluctua-
tions of the capillary oxygen tension and the oxygen delivery
to tissues. There is an adaptation by an increase of the
tissue flow, when either tissue oxygen demand increases or
the possibility of oxygen delivery decreases. In recent
years it has been shown, that the availability of oxygen
in patients with diabetes mellitus depends on the degree
of metabolic control. A shift of the oxygen dissociation
curve of oxyhemoglobin and elevated levels of hemoglobin
components with an increased affinity to oxygen are the
main factors in the development of tissue hypoxia in patients with diabetes mellitus.

A fall of the oxygen tension (Po_2) results in a decreased
saturation of hemoglobin for oxygen and the release of oxygen
to the tissues. A decreased pH as occurs in the peripheral
tissues, causes a rightward shift in the curve (decreased
affinity of hemoglobin for oxygen, Bohr's effect), facilitating a greater release of oxygen. An increase of the carbon

dioxide tension (Pco_2) and an increased intraerythrocytic concentration of 2-3-diphosphoglyceric acid (2-3 D.P.G.) also shifts the oxyhemoglobin dissociation curve to the right. When the oxygen tension falls, a decreased pH, an increased Pco_2 and an increased 2-3 D.P.G. concentration in the erythrocyte stimulate the release of oxygen to the tissues. A rise of the pH, a fall of the Pco_2 and a decrease of the 2-3 D.P.G. concentration have the opposite effect. The normal oxyhemoglobin dissociation curve is shown in the figure.

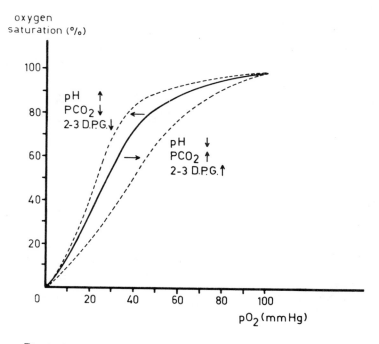

Fig: 1 The influence of the pH, PCO_2 and 2-3 D.P.G. on the oxygen dissociation curve of oxyhemoglobin.

143

The 2-3 D.P.G. in the red cell is generated by anaerobic glycolysis of glucose. Increased levels of 2-3 D.P.G. have been found in a variety of conditions with evidence of hypoxic stress such as high altitude exposure, hypoxemia from congenital heart disease and pulmonary insufficiency. In diabetes the 2-3 D.P.G. concentration of the red cell depends on metabolic changes. A blood pH below normal and a lowering of the concentration of plasma inorganic phosphate lead to an inhibition in the formation of 2-3 D.P.G. in the red cell (Ditzel and Standl 1975). Both changes are of importance in ketoacidosis and result in a decreased release of oxygen from oxyhemoglobin for several days after the recovery from the acidosis. The normalization of the 2-3 D.P.G. concentration of the erythrocyte takes some days. Repeated acidotic dysregulation in diabetic patients therefore coincides with periods of decreased oxygen release and tissue hypoxia. Increased levels of hemoglobin components with a high oxygen affinity also contribute to the development of tissue hypoxia in diabetes mellitus (Paulsen and Koury 1976). These components of normal hemoglobin A are fast moving in a chromatographic system and are indicated as HbA_{1a}, HbA_{1b} and HbA_{1c}. They differ from normal hemoglobin A by having a hexose bound to the B-chain of hemoglobin. Normally the three hemoglobin components comprise about 7 percent of total hemoglobin. The major component is HbA_{1c}, where glucose is bound to the aminogroup of the B-chain. The blocking of the aminogroup greatly reduces the reactivity of hemoglobin with 2-3 D.P.G. resulting in a hemoglobin with high affinity for oxygen. In situations where blood glucose levels are increased like in diabetes mellitus glycosylation is stimulated resulting in increased HbA_1 levels. HbA_{1c} concentration being normally about 5 percent of total hemoglobin may increase to 15 percent in patients with diabetes mellitus. Therefore elevated blood glucose levels contribute directly to the development of tissue hypoxia in diabetes mellitus. Increased levels of HbA_1 persist in the diabetic for a considerable time after ketoacidosis is corrected. Good control gradually represses the HbA_1 concentrations to normal in the course of one to two months. Estimation of the HbA_1 concentration therefore is a good measure of diabetic control during the previous weeks.

Besides the decreased availability of oxygen by a lack of 2-3 D.P.G. and an increase of HbA_1 in poorly controlled patients with diabetes mellitus, a disturbed peripheral circulation plays a role in the development of tissue hypoxia in diabetes mellitus. An increase in plasma viscosity, a more pronounced intravascular red cell and thrombocytes aggregation and a decreased fibrinolysis contribute to the disturbed peripheral circulation. All these factors contribute to the development of microangiopathy.

The process of glycosylation of the aminogroup of proteins, as discussed for hemoglobin, also seems to hold true for proteins of the basal membrane. In that case glucose has a direct damaging effect. Such a relationship exists most obviously in microvascular disease of the kidney. In the diabetic animal an increased activity in the kidney of the enzyme glycosyl transferase, which could lead to a carbohydrate-rich membrane has been reported. Normalization of the blood glucose levels in these animals by careful insulin treatment restores the glucosyltransferase content to normal (Spiro and Spiro 1971, Spiro 1976). In the glomerular basal membrane of diabetic patients an increased glucose content has been found. All these data make it probable, that thickening of the basal membrane occurs as a result of metabolic disturbances. Besides that the alterations of the basal membrane increase with the duration of the diabetic state (Kilo e.a. 1972).

Thickening of the capillary basement membrane is not an irreversible condition, which follows from the regression of the basal membrane thickening in animal experiments after successful transplantation of islets of Langerhans or the whole pancreas. Transplantation of kidneys of diabetic rats in normal rats gives a regression or even a disappearance of the characteristic microangiopathy. The reverse also has been described. Microangiopathy appears when normal kidneys are transplanted in diabetic rats (Matas 1976). All these experiments indicate, that it is possible to prevent microangiopathic alterations or to treat them by normalization of the blood glucose levels.

Thickening of the capillary basement membrane seems also not to be an irreversible condition in the human. Normalization of the triglyceride levels in patients with hypertriglyceridemia coincides with a decrease in basal membrane thickness (De Vries e.a. 1974). Hypertriglyceridemia occurs frequently in patients with diabetes mellitus. It may result from an increased synthesis and/or a decreased removal of triglycerides. Reaven e.a. showed that the rise in triglycerides after administering a carbohydrate-rich diet is associated with the height of the insulin levels (1967). On the other hand, it is known, that there is a defect in the removal of triglycerides in patients with diabetes. Insulin deficiency coincides with a decreased plasma heparin lipolytic activity, as can be shown by a 5 hour heparin infusion. A disturbed equilibrium of triglyceride synthesis and removal causes hypertriglyceridemia in diabetes mellitus of the overweight type. Hypertriglyceridemia as such seems

146

of importance for the development of microvascular disease and atherosclerosis. Extreme hypertriglyceridemia resulting in a milky turbulance of the plasma depresses oxygen release from oxyhemoglobin and disturbs the microcirculation (Ditzel and Dyerberg 1977). A correlation between serum triglyceride levels and the concentration of HbA_{1c} has also been demonstrated (Peterson e.a. 1977).

Other late diabetic complications, which seem to coincide with a disturbed glucose metabolism are: increased kidney tubular glycogen storage, the occurrence of a cataract of the lens and diabetic neuropathy. Neuropathy and cataract are based on a stimulation of the so-called polyol pathway. With decreased insulin activity and hyperglycemia glucose is independent from insulin converted to sorbitol and fructose (Gabbay 1973). Storage of these products in the Schwann cells seems to be of importance in the development of diabetic neuropathy. Correction of the hyperglycemia results in an improvement of the nerve conduction in the early phase of neuropathy (Ward e.a. 1971).

Based on the above mentioned data the American Diabetes Association recently made the statement, that microvascular complications decrease by reduction of blood glucose concentrations (Cahill e.a. 1976). The same holds true for early diabetic neuropathy. The goal of treatment therefore should be to keep blood sugar levels during the major part of the day below a level of 200 mg/dl. (11 mmol/l.). To achieve this a more physiologic way of insulin administration should be strived after. The development of an artificial pancreas, which delivers insulin immediately when glucose levels rise, offers the possibility to achieve normal glucose levels during the 24-48 hours, when the patient is connected with the apparatus. The delivery of insulin from the artificial pancreas gives a rough impression of the pattern of insulin substitution, which the patient needs.

This means that when single daily insulin injections do not lead to acceptable regulation of the blood glucose level, multiple daily injections are preferable. Actually only those patients, who have sufficient endogenous insulin reserve to catch up the glucose rise after meals, can be treated with one daily injection of insulin. Patients without any endogenous insulin production need multiple daily injections of insulin, dependent on their meals. As multiple daily injections are not possible from the patient's point of view, a compromise has to be sought, e.g. two daily injections of intermediate-acting insulin. If one succeeds by the use of divided doses of insulin to improve diabetic control, also the progression of already existing diabetic retinopathy is decreased (Job e.a. 1976). The relationship between the metabolic control of diabetes and the occurrence of retinopathy was recently confirmed in animal experiments with alloxan-diabetic dogs (Engerman e.a. 1977). Against the background that diabetic retinopathy is the second cause of blindness, better control of diabetes is an important goal.

A special problem form those patients who have diabetes and an extreme overweight. The main cause of hyperglycemia in these patients is the resistance to the peripheral action of insulin. As judged from the high insulin levels which are reached after a meal, insulin reserve in these patients would be sufficient if they lose enough weight. Exogenous insuline administration is not very effective in overweight diabetic patients and besides that not advisable, as this treatment contributes to a further increase of body-weight. Considerable weight loss mostly results in an important lowering or even normalization of the blood glucose levels. Therefore in these patients the achievement of a normal body weight by prescribing a low caloric diet without oral antidiabetic agents or insulin substitution remains the best treatment.

Literature

1. Cahill, G.F., Erzwiler, D.D. and Freinkel, N. (1976): Blood glucose control in diabetes. Diabetes 25, 237.
2. Danowski, T.S., Fisher, E.R., Khurana, R.C., Nolan, S. and Stephan, T. (1972): Muscle capillary basement membrane in juvenile diabetes mellitus. Metabolism 21, 1125.
3. Ditzel, J. and Dyerberg, J. (1977): Hyperlipoproteinemia, diabetes and oxygen affinity of hemoglobin. Metabolism 26, 141.
4. Ditzel, J. and Standl, E. (1975): The problem of tissue oxygenation in diabetes mellitus. Act. Med. Scand. Suppl. 578, 49, 59, 69.
5. Engerman, R., Bloodworth, J.M.B. and Nelson, S. (1977): Relationship in microvascular disease in diabetes to metabolic control. Diabetes 26, 760.
6. Gabbay, K.H. (1973): The sorbitol pathway and the complications of diabetes. New Engl. J. Med. 288, 831.
7. Job, D., Eschwege, E., Guyot-Argenton, C., Aubrey, J.P. and Tchobroutsky, G. (1976): The effect of multiple daily insulin injections in the course of diabetic retinopathy. Diabetes 25, 463.

8. Jordan, S.W. and Perley, M.J. (1972): Microangiopathy in diabetes mellitus and aging. Arch. Path. 93, 261.

9. Kilo, C., Vogler, N. and Williamson, J.R. (1972): Muscle capillary basement membrane changes related to aging and diabetes mellitus. Diabetes 21, 881.

10. Matas, A.J., Sutherland, D.E.R. and Najarian, J.S. (1976): Current status of islet and pancreas transplantation in diabetes. Diabetes 25, 785.

11. Paulsen E. and Doury, M. (1976): Hemoglobin A_{1c} levels in insulin dependent and -independent diabetes mellitus. Diabetes 25, Suppl. 2, 890.

12. Peterson, C.M., Koenig, R.J., Jones, R.L., Saudeh, C.D. and Cerami, C. (1977): Correlation of serum triglyceride levels and hemoglobin A_{1c} concentrations in diabetes mellitus. Diabetes 26, 507.

13. Reaven, G.M., Lerner, R.L., Stern, M.P. and Farquhar, J.W. (1967): Role of insulin in endogenous hypertriglyceridemia. J. Clin. Invest. 46, 1756.

14. Siperstein, M.D., Unger, R.H. and Madison, L.L. (1968): Studies of muscle capillary basement membranes in normal subjects, diabetic and prediabetic subjects. J. Clin. Invest. 47, 1973.

15. Spiro, R.G. (1976): Investigations into the biochemical basis of diabetic basement membrane alterations. Diabetes 25, Suppl. 2, 909.

16. Spiro, R.G. and Spiro, M.J. (1971): Effect of diabetes on the biosynthesis of the renal glomerular basement membrane. Studies on the glucosyltransferase. Diabetes 20, 641.

17. De Vries, O., Vos, J., Reitsma, W.D., Doorenbos, H. and Molenaar, I. (1974): Muscular capillary basement membrane hypertrophy in hyperlipaemia type IV: a reversible consequence of a metabolic disorder? Neth. J. of Med. 17, 220.

18. Ward, J.D., Barnes, C.G., Fisher, D.J., Jessop, J.D. and Baker, R.W.R. (1971): Improvement in nerve conduction following treatment in newly diagnosed diabetics. Lancet 1, 428.

19. Williamson, J.R. and Kilo, C. (1977): Current status of capillary basement membrane disease in diabetes mellitus. Diabetes 26, 65.

CHAPTER XV
ORAL ANTIDIABETIC DRUGS AND CARDIOVASCULAR COMPLICATIONS
Saleh, A.E.C.

Since in 1970 the University Group Diabetes Program
(U.G.D.P.) (1970, 1975) published the results of their prospective study on the efficacy of various modes of diabetic
treatment, in postponing the appearance or delaying the
progression of vascular complications, a great debate has
been raised on the important subject concerning hypoglyce
mic therapy with oral antidiabetic drugs. This discussion
is currently one of the most controversial issues in medicine. Therefore it seems very opportune to bring this matter up at this course. Maybe together then we can formulate
a workable conclusion to help those of us who have to guide
their diabetic patients and are obliged to choose one or
other therapeutic regimen.

In 1961 a cooperative prospective clinical trial was
started by 12 medical centres in the United States of
America. One thousand twenty seven (1027) patients were admitted to the study; 71% were females and 54% were white
people. All subjects belonged to the group of maturity onset diabetes, non insulin dependent, diagnosed within one
year of admission to the study. They were arbitrary judged
by the physicians at the various centres to have a life
expectancy of at least five years.

Patients were assigned randomly to five different
treatment groups. All received a diet adapted to their

weight and beside this *group I* 205 patients received a placebo, *group II* 204 patients received a fixed dose of 1500 mg tolbutamide, *group III* 210 patients were given a fixed dose of insulin (10 to 16 U Insulin Lente^R) according to their body surface, *group IV* 204 patients recieved an insulin dose adapted to variation of their glycemia. The last *group V* 204 patients used a fixed dose of phenformin 100 mg daily.

At quarterly intervals every patient was reviewed and had a general examination with special attention to their glucoregulation, ocular, cardiac, renal and peripheral vascular condition. No changes were brought in their treatment except in group IV and if there was an absolute indication for one or other reason that might endanger the patients life. If a patient died an internist and a pathologist determined the cause of death.

The mortality results of the study were rather shocking. The highest percentages of deaths were found in the groups treated with either tolbutamide (14,7%) or phenformin (16,7%). These percentages were for the placebogroup, and the groups with a fixed or a variable dose of insulin respectively 10,2%, 9,5% and 8,5%. These statistically not significant higher mortality rates in the groups of patients treated with oral hypoglycemic agents proved to be caused by a statistically significant higher death rate by cardiovascular causes. Cardiovascular mortality was in the placebo group 4,9%, in the fixed insulin dose group 6,2%, in the variable insulin dose group 5,9%, in the tolbutamide group 12,7% and in the phenformin group 13,2%.

The United States Food and Drug Administration, the American Diabetic Association (although in guarded terms) and the American Medical Association endorsed these assertions, therefore the use of tolbutamide in 1969 and of phenformin in 1971 has been discontinued. It was recommended that oral antidiabetic drugs should be used only as a last resort in patients who cannot be controlled by diet or weight loss and for whom the addition of insulin is impracticable or unacceptable.

Other prospective studies done in a rather similar way and with the same purpose are at variance with those reported by the U.G.D.P.

Keen (1971) studied in Bedford England 132 men and 116 women with borderline diabetes and mean ages respectively 55.4 and 58.9 years. The treatment consisted of 1 gram of tolbutamide or a placebo.

After seven years of treatment there were 25 death in the placebo group of which 14 were cardiovascular cases. For the tolbutamide group the numbers were 24 deaths of which 12 cardiovascular. So there was no difference at all.

Paasikivi (1971) treated 178 non diabetic patients, survivors of a single infarction with a placebo or tolbutamide (dose 750 or 1000 mg). The survival rate of the tolbutamide treated patients improved significantly over 1½ to 2 years as compared with that of the control group, although in later years this advantage was lost and the difference between the two groups disappeared.

Feldman (1974) studied 350 asymptomatic diabetics between the ages of 15 and 59 years. They were randomly treated with tolbutamide 1 gram daily, phenformin 100 mg daily or placebo. The results covering about 8 years of observation showed only 1 cardiovascular death and 8 non cardiovascular accidents of which 3 in the tolbutamide group, 3 in the phenformin group and 2 in the placebo group. So no difference was found.

Of all the above mentioned studies one can say that although the maximum effort was made to diminish as much as possible the cause of errors normally attached to randomised trials, still certain factors were more frequent especially in the U.G.D.P. group at the start of the study in the tolbutamide treated group. However, this fact has been incalculated in the sophisticated statistical work-up of the findings.

The U.G.D.P.-study has been criticized by many clinicians. To solve the controversery a commission of the biometric society was instituted to reassess the U.G.D.P. data. The judgment of the commission can best be summarized by quoting some of their conclusions. (Report of the Committee for the assessment of biometric aspects of controlled trials of hypoglycemic agents (1975)):

"On the question of cardiovascular mortality due to tolbutamide and phenformin, we consider that the U.G.D.P. trial has raised suspicions that cannot be dismissed on the basis of other evidence presently available. We find most of the criticism levelled against the U.G.D.P. findings on this point unpersuasive. The possibility that deaths may have been allocated to cardiovascular causes preferentially in the groups receiving oral therapy exists, and, in view of the "non-significance" of differences in total mortality, some reservation about the conclusion that the oral hypoglycemics are toxic must remain. Nonetheless, we consider the evidence of harmfulness moderately strong. -In conclusion, we consider that in the light of the U.G.D.P. findings, it remains with the proponents of the oral hypoglycemics to conduct scientifically adequate studies to justify the continued use of such agents".

Some recent studies give more insight in the mechanism

by which oral hypoglycemic agents might damage the heart.

Insulin is known to have a positive inotropic effect on the heart. Also tolbutamide augments the contractility of the heart in rabbits and cats but not in dogs. There are studies that support a positive inotropic effect on the human heart. A significant increase in the frequency of ventricular fibrillation among diabetics on oral hypoglycemic drugs has been reported (Levey e.a. 1974).

This is not known of phenformin, however, it is known that phenformin increases both the systolic and diastolic blood pressure and also increases the heart rate (U.G.D.P. 1975). This effect might be nocive for the heart especially if this is already damaged. A report of increased frequency of myocarditis and visceral microgranuloma in 29 patients treated with tolbutamide has not been confirmed. (Editorial, 1971).

In conclusion we may say that keeping a balanced diet with the goal of reaching a normal body weight is the first choice of treatment in maturity onset diabetes. If this is not successful and the patient loses too much weight and remains glucosuric, insulin substitution is needed. Only in those maturity onset diabetics, in whom insulin substitution is difficult to realize for practical reasons and diet alone is not sufficiently effective, sulfonyl ureum derivatives like tolbutamide or glibenclamide may be indicated. Biguanides induce beside a possible increased risk for cardiovascular mortality a higher incidence of lactic acidosis. In fact the latter drugs like phenformin should no longer be prescribed (Williams and Palmer, 1975).

References

1. Editorial, (1971): Lancet 1, 171.
2. Feldman, R., Crawford, D., Elashoff, R. and Glass, A.
   (1974): Oral hypoglycemic drug prophylaxis in asymptomatic diabetes. Diabetes, Proceedings of the eighth
   Congress of the I.D.F., 574. Editors: W.J. Malaisse,
   J. Pirart and J. Vallance Owen. Excerpta Medica, Amsterdam.
3. Keen, H. (1971): Factors influencing the progress of
   atherosclerosis in the diabetic. Acta diab. lat. 8,
   Suppl. 1, 444.
4. Levey, G.S., Lasseter, K.C. and Palmer, R.F. (1974):
   Sulfonylureas and the heart. Ann. Rev. Med. 25, 69.
5. Paasikivi, J. (1970): Long-term tolbutamide treatment
   after myocardial infarction. A clinical and biochemical
   study of 178 patients without overt diabetes. Acta med.
   scand. 187, Suppl. 507, 1.
6. Report of the Committee for the assessment of biometric
   aspects of the controlled trials of hypoglycemic agents.
   (1975). J. Amer. med. Ass. 231, 583.
7. University Group Diabetes Program (1970 and 1975): A
   study of the effects of hypoglycemic agents on vascular
   complications in patients with adult-onset diabetes.
   Diabetes 19, Suppl. 2, 747 and Diabetes 24, Suppl. 1, 65.
8. Williams, R.H. and Palmer, J.P. (1975): Farewell to phenformin for treating diabetes mellitus. Ann. of Int. Med.
   83, 567.

CHAPTER XVI
ATHEROSCLEROSIS AND THE PEDIATRICIAN

Winkel, C.A.

There is a growing conviction that the only way to substantially reduce the toll from atherosclerotic disease, is to attack its constitutional and environmental precursors long before overt symptoms occur. In 1965 Reisman called for possible pediatric responsibility in the prophylaxis of atherosclerosis (1). The apparent progression from fatty streak to fibrous plaque and the substantial increments in these changes in middle to late childhood and again in the second to third decade of life, has been demonstrated (2-5). It was apparent from the early data that many atherosclerotic lesions reached a presumably irreversible stage in the third decade of life.

Atherosclerosis in the human aorta is probably universally present in all populations by 3 years of age and is found somewhat later in the coronary arteries in children in populations where the disease is prevalent in the adult.

A number of epidemiologic studies have identified certain risk factors, such as elevated serum cholesterol, elevated bloodpressure, diminished carbohydrate tolerance, smoking of cigarettes, emotional stress and decreased physical fitness leading to disease and it has been shown that a combination of these is more detrimental than each occurring singly. Most of these risk factors can be ascribed to faulty living habits and it is assumed that these could be corrected if sufficient consideration is taken with genetic, cultural and environmental factors influencing rise and consequent development of cardiovascular disease due to atherosclerosis.

A risk factor is a personal characteristic which is associated with an excessive rate of development of overt disease. The causality of these factors depends upon evidence resulting from animal experiments, metabolic studies on humans, and pathology found at death.

Whether it will help to correct risk factors requires a clinical trial in which these factors are modified. Modifying risk factors in adults has thus far not been an unequivocal success. Aside from the positive influence achieved by control of hypertension and the giving up of cigarette smoking; other changes such as diet modifications by lowering lipids in middle age with the purpose of delaying atherosclerotic cardiovascular disease, have been inconclusive and largely disappointing.

Some think that there are little convincing data which show that attention to risk factors in adults in fact prolong their life, and conclude that it is premature to recommend preventive measures for children. Lack of success in adults may be a reason for even more emphasis on a preventive program for children. After all, measures begun late in life to alter the precursors of disease, a process which has been going on for decades and is in a stage in which lesions are well advanced; may not be effective. We cannot expect measures taken in these circumstances in the relative short time of a clinical trial, to have any effect.

If the genesis of atherosclerosis is in childhood, identification of a subset of the pediatric population at high risk for atherosclerosis might make an approach to primary prevention of cardiovascular disease possible. One approach to primary prevention of cardiovascular disease might begin by identifying children with elevated levels of cholesterol, triglycerides or both.

In several population studies done in schoolchildren and using 215 to 230 mg% of cholesterol as an upper limit for normal, a considerable number were found to have modest elevation of cholesterol (8,9,10,11,12,14). Some of these studies coincided with autopsy findings which suggested that apparent precursors of mature atherosclerotic plaque might be detected in childhood (13). The cholesterol concentration in the neonate is approximately 65 mg/100 ml during the first months of life. Later on cholesterol concentration rises, reaching a mean value of 165 mg/100 ml by 2 years. There is no further significant variation in cholesterol with age, sex, rate of growth or level of sexual maturation until approximately 20 years of age. At that time a slow progressive rise begins that continues until about 60 years (6-7).

Cholesterol concentration of the neonate is approximately 1/3 that of maternal blood. The fetus is nourished on a very low fat diet. The primary nutritional sources for the fetus are aminoacids, glucose and small amounts of fatty acids. Placental transport of cholesterol and triglycerides is minimal. Soon after birth a diet high in calories, cholesterol and saturated fats is introduced with human milk.

Familial hypercholesterolemia and familial hypertriglyceridemia should be ruled out and differentiated from hypercholesterolemia and hypertriglyceridemia secondary to dietary excess. As the first are statistically heir to

atherosclerosis, kindreds with early morbid or lethal coronary vascular disease should be ascertained and serum
lipids and serum lipoproteins in children from these kindreds systematically analysed.

Dietary management which has a substantial role in
the long term management of familial hypercholesterolemia
and hypertriglyceridemia in childhood, should be instituted.
Whether normalization of elevated cholesterol and triglyceride levels in children with inherited or acquired hyper-
lipidemias will reduce the substantial risk of premature
atherosclerosis in later life, is not yet known.

A good case can be made for periodic blood cholesterol
monitoring,for diet and weight control in *all* children with
values exceeding 180 mg% (depending of normal cholesterol
for age in population): and also in children of families
with premature atherosclerosis with or without demonstrable
lipid metabolic defect.

Most atherogenic diseases, according to most research-
ers, do not evolve from people with inborn error of lipid
metabolism, but arise from a segment of the population with
more moderate lipid elevation, although some conditions represent a heterozygous error of lipid metabolism, most with
moderate elevation result from faulty diet and positive
energy balance.

In the Netherlands-Antilles food habits have been
changing during the last 15 years. As very little food is
produced on the islands, most food products are imported and
the daily diet has become very much like the diet in the
United States. Foods rich in carbohydrates, saturated fats
and cholesterol, made their entry available in numerous
snackbars, ice-cream and pizza parlors and in the younger
age group, the infant gets the same brands of milk and the

same type of babyfood as are available in the USA, so that the dietary risk factors of acquiring atherosclerotic vascular heart disease show the same pattern as in the Western countries.

The *smoking* habit is acquired early in life and is more early established in adolescents, exposed to it by their peers and parents. Cigarette consumption in boys and girls is increasing in the Netherlands-Antilles. Cigarette smoking is a little threat to cardiovascular health in young adolescents. The toll is exacted later after the habit has become tenaciously established and the cardiovascular system becomes more vulnerable to its effect. As the impact of the nicotine habit is greatest in the young, particularly the more so with raised cholesterol and bloodpressure levels. The inception of smoking in the child is related to smoking in the parent. Parent and teacher ought to give the good example by not smoking. It should be appreciated that as with other educational endeavours health related behaviour can be most effectly be influenced by lessons learned early in life.

Obesity is associated with hypertriglyceridemia and diabetes mellitus and is in this way an indirect risk factor associated with angina pectoris and myocardial infarction.

"Does the fat infant become the fat adult?"

The concept of a fat infant developing in a fat adult has become increasingly attractive with the advent of reports on the growth of the adipose cells, first in number and then in size. Adults who where fat in childhood developed a larger number of fat cells than adults whose obesity developed later. The later had enlarged fat cells,

162

though a normal number of them. This increased number of
fat cells is thought to be permanent and may be a potent
factor in the continuation of later obesity.

The etiology of the abnormal positive energy balance
producing caloric retention may be either inactivity or
excessive caloric intake, possibly relating to faulty eating
or sedentary living patterns. Weight gain in early life
appears related to the weight pattern in later life, either
by provoking resistant hyperplastic obesity or a tenacious
pattern of overeating by alteration in food control mechanisms. Sound information on nutrition should be given to
the parents. Breastfeeding should be encouraged, delay in
use of solid foods in infancy (4-6 months), emphasis on
eating behaviour, rather than diets should be stressed.
Nutrient excess discouraged.

Hypertension is one of the most common and potent elements predisposing to coronary disease. Hypertension clearly tends to run in the family. Genetic factors assist in
identifying the population at risk i.c. family history of
hypertension, myocardial infarction or stroke.

Salt intake is likely to be one of the environmental
contributing factors for those whose genetic make-up predisposes them to hypertension. There is evidence in rats
relating hypertension to salt intake. Strains of rats have
been raised by Dahl that are highly salt sensitive; when
they are salt fed early in life, they are made hypertensive (14). Primitive societies on low salt intake do not
show the progressive rise in blood pressure as seen in our
society, so that this phenomenon cannot be considered unavoidable or physiologic.

The consumption of "presalted" foods may be producing
significant changes in salt intake in our society which

are not perceived at this time. The question whether a documentated level of arterial pressure in an infant or child is predictive of the level in that individual as an adult, remains to be answered. It has been suggested that a childs blood pressure remains at a relatively fixed place in the blood pressure distribution curve of the general population for age and sex throughout childhood and into adolescence and adult life. This phenomenon referred to as "tracking", implies that if blood pressure at a certain young age is at the 50th percentile, it will remain at the 50th percentile, unless influenced by disease factors, affecting blood pressure control. Preliminary statistical longitudinal data suggest that tracking is present from early childhood. How early in life this is of sufficient significance to be clinically useful remains to be determined (15,16). So it appears that the best predictor of later hypertension is the level of blood pressure at some earlier date, as in childhood or its presence in the parents.

Overweight and heart rate have been observed to make modest independent contribution to the risk of hypertension developing in children. These observations, though requiring further study, lend support to the possibility that relatively simple hygienic measures, such as control of weight and avoidance of salt intake, may have great potential for primary prevention of hypertension in those identified as being at increased risk at an early age.

Summarizing we may say that the pediatrician in his role of health maintenance can alter the appalling cardio-vascular mortality statistics by not allowing the process or the habits and conditions which promote it to become firmly established and irreversible.

Cardiovascular disease begins in childhood with what may be regarded as medical trivia such as a tendency to obesity, moderate serum lipid, and blood pressure elevations, lack of exercise and the cigarette habit. We must establish goals based on optimal as distinct from average levels of blood pressure, bloodlipids and weight.

Prevention of atherosclerosis is a family affair which must include the children as well as the parents.

References:

1. Reisman, M. (1965): J. Pediat. 66, 1.
2. Enos, W.F. et al. (1953): J.A.M.A. 152, 1090.
3. Strong, J.P. et al. (1969): J. Atheroscler. Res. 9, 251.
4. McMillan, G.C. (1973): Am. J. Cardiol. 31, 542.
5. McNamara, J.J. et al. (1971): J.A.M.A. 216, 1185.
6. Glueck, C.J. et al. (1971): Metabolism 20, 597.
7. Clarke, R.P. et al. (1970): Am. J. Clin. Nutr. 23, 745.
8. Hodges, R.E. et al. (1965): Am. J. Clin. Nutr. 17, 200.
9. Golubjatnikov, R. et al. (1972): Am. J. Epidem. 96, 36.
10. Godfrey, R.G. et al. (1972): Aust. Paediat. J. 8, 72.
11. Duplessis, J.P. et al. (1967): S.A. Med. J. 41, 1216.
12. Starr, P. (1971): Am. J. Clin. Path. 56, 515.
13. Vlodaver, Z. et al. (1969): Circulation 39, 541.
14. Dahl, L.K. et al. (1968): Circulation Res. 22, 11.
15. Miall, W.E. et al. (1967): Br. Med. J. 2, 660.
16. Zinner, S.H. et al. (1971): N. Engl. J. Med. 284, 401.

CHAPTER XVII
DIAGNOSIS AND TREATMENT OF PERIPHERAL
ATHEROSCLEROTIC DISEASE

Nieveen, J., Wouda, A.A., Bernink, P.J.L.M.
Groningen, The Netherlands

INTRODUCTION

Atherosclerotic narrowing or occlusion of peripheral arteries is often the cause of much complaining and suffering of these patients.

In contradiction to patients with angina pectoris and myocardial infarction, the mortality in this group of patients is less, but many people are handicapped by atherosclerotic disease of the peripheral arteries in the legs. Peripheral artery disease of the arms is of very minor importance. This lecture therefore will be confined to atherosclerotic disease of the legs.

According to the Netherland Central Organisation for Statistics in 1971-1972 $\pm$ 70.300 persons were disabled by peripheral vascular diseases in comparison to $\pm$ 38.600 patients with cerebrovascular lesions.

Symptoms of peripheral atherosclerosis

The narrowing of peripheral arteries of the legs can give two different types of symptoms:
1) intermittent claudication, caused by diminished muscle circulation
2) skinlesions caused by diminished skin circulation

1) Intermittent claudication

Dependent on the site of the artery lesion pain in the
muscles of the hip (a. iliaca communis) - of the upperleg
(in case of narrowing of the external iliac artery) - or
pain in the calfs (narrowing of the femoral arteries) can
occur. This pain has a cramping character and occurs during
exercise. The walking distance is a measure for the serious-
ness of the arterial narrowing.

2) Skin lesions

The most important symptoms are coldness of the feet,
calcified nails, less growing of the nails, loss of hairgrowth on the feet, bad healing of wounds, ulcera and in
the terminal stage gangrene of the foot.

DIAGNOSTIC PROCEDURES

General examination

Of course atherosclerotic lesions should be differentiated from neurological-arthrotic-rheumatical diseases
and general examination is necessary in order to detect
other diseases for instance angina pectoris, cerebrovascular
diseases, hypertension, diabetes, hyperlipoproteinemias,
external riskfactors as smoking cigarettes, overweight and
so on.

Treatment of these diseases and symptoms is of course
necessary together with the specific treatment of the peripheral vascular disease.

General examination of the legs

Inspection shows the condition of the skin (atrophy, hairgrowth, nails, wounds a.s.o.). *Palpation* gives an impression of the skintemperature and of the pulsations of the *abdominal aorta* (near the umbilicus), of the *femoral arteries* (in the inguinal region), the *popliteal arteries* (in the hollow of the knee), the *posterior tibial arteries* (at the back of the inner malleolus) and the *dorsal pedis arteries* (at the dorsum of the feet). To exclude cerebrovascular and armartery lesions it is also necessary to palpate the carotid, subclavian, radial and ulnar arteries.

Auscultation

When arteries are narrowed more than $\pm$ 50 %, systolic murmurs can be heard below the site of the narrowing.

To get an impression of the skincirculation, Ratschow described a simple test: The patient is in horizontal position, the legs vertical. He is moving his feet during one minute 40-60 times. In case of arterial insufficiency the skin of the foot and toes becomes white. Then the patient is placed in sitting position with the legs hanging downwards. Normally in between 5 seconds a reactive hyperaemia of the toes is seen (capillary flush).

In case of arterial insufficiency the occurrence of reactive hyperaemia comes later. Also a measure of the arterial circulation is the filling time of the veins on the back of the feet. Normally filling is seen 10 seconds after taking the sitting position. In arterial lesions this fillingtime lasts longer (> 20 sec).

Claudication time

Most accurately and objectively claudication time is
measured with the help of a treadmill. We use a speed of
3,6 km/hr, (= 60 m/min, or 1 m/sec and walking uphill 6°.

As an example the data of a patient 50 years of age,
are sampled on the scheme (Fig. 1).

The arteries of the left leg could not be palpated,
claudication time (in the calf) was 200 meter, a type IV
hyperlipoproteinaemia and a disturbed glucose tolerance
test was found. The patient smoked 25 cigarettes per day.
There was an overweight (85.5 kg, length 1.76 m).

More specialized diagnostic methods

A. Oscillography

The volume changes of arms and legs caused by the
arterial pulsations are transferred to bloodpressure cuffs.
With the oscillograph one registrates the changes in pressure in the cuffs. The measurements are performed at both
legs at the same time and the results compared. The cuffs
should be positioned at equal sites at both legs (upper
and calfs). The cuffs are inflated to a pressure of
250 mmHg. Every time after registration of 4-5 pulses, the
pressure is reduced stepwise with 25 mmHg, till the pressure is only 25 mmHg. With this method qualitative differences of the maximal pulse amplitudes in both legs can be
found and so an indication can be given of a narrowing of
arteries in the legs. Figure 2 shows the oscillo gram of
the described patient. A clear difference between right
upper leg and left upper leg is shown.

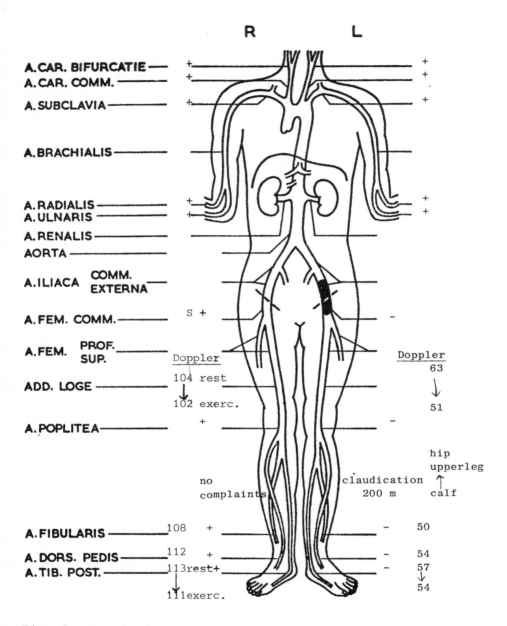

R   L

A.CAR. BIFURCATIE ——   +   +
A.CAR. COMM. ———   +   +
A.SUBCLAVIA ———   +   +

A.BRACHIALIS ———

A.RADIALIS ———   +   +
A.ULNARIS ———   +   +
A.RENALIS ———
AORTA ———

A.ILIACA COMM. EXTERNA ———

A.FEM. COMM. ———   S +   —

A.FEM. PROF. SUP. ———

       Doppler   Doppler
       104 rest   63
ADD. LOGE ———   ↓   ↓
       102 exerc.   51

A.POPLITEA ———   +   —

                            hip
                            upperleg
    no   claudication   ↑
    complaints   200 m   calf

A.FIBULARIS ———   108 +   — 50
A.DORS. PEDIS ———   112 +   — 54
A.TIB. POST. ———   113rest+   — 57
                               ↓
       111exerc.   54

Fig. 1. See text.

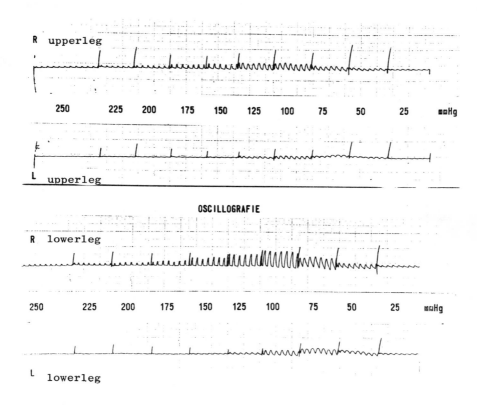

Fig. 2.   See text.

B. Photoelectric plethysmography

    With the photoelectric plethysmogram (FEP) the blood-
volume changes in skinvessels can be demonstrated (Elings,
1959; De Pater et al., 1962). As oscillography this method
is also a qualitative one. A scattereye is placed on the
toes, and/or fingers of the patients. This element com-
prises a light source and a Light Dependent Resistance
(LDR) element. The light falling on the skin is mostly

absorbed by the blood, partly scattered and partly reflected. The larger the bloodcontent of the skinvessels,
the less light is reflected. The resistence of the LDR
element changes with the amount of reflected light. These
changes can be recorded with an electrocardiograph and so
bloodvolume curves of the skinvessels can be obtained.
Fig. 3 shows schematically the element.

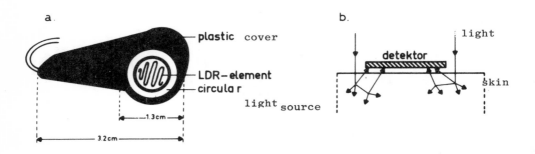

Fig. 3. Photoelectric plethysmography.

In order to exclude spastic conditions of the small
skinvessels, the legs of the patients are placed for 30
minutes under a hot box. After this period the curves are
recorded. In case of obliterations in the larger arteries,
the FEP curve will be abnormal (lower amplitude, convexity
in stead of concavity of the descending limb of the curve).
Fig. 4 shows the FEP after hot box of our patient (paperspeed 25 mm/sec).

C. It is also possible to get an objective measurement of
the reactive *hyperaemia* with the aid of the FEP. The FEP
is recorded with a paperspeed of 0.25 mm/sec. During 2
minutes the arterial circulation of the legs is occluded

172

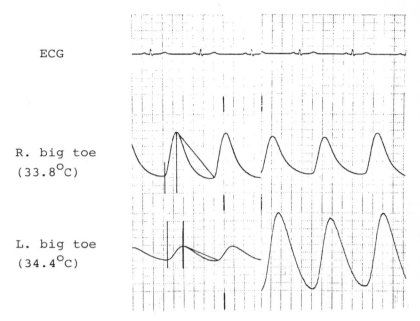

Fig. 4. Photoelectric plethysmogram after hot box from described patient. Sensitivity right lower curve 5x as large as other curves.

by inflating a cuff around the upper leg, above 250 mmHg. After 2 minutes this pressure is suddenly stopped and a reactive hyperaemia is recorded.

Normally the pulsations reappear immediately after stopping the pressure. The amplitudes are higher than before, coming down gradually to the original height. In pathological circumstances there exists a latent period, the amplitudes are not high and come only slightly back to their original size. Fig. 5 shows the curves of the described patient.

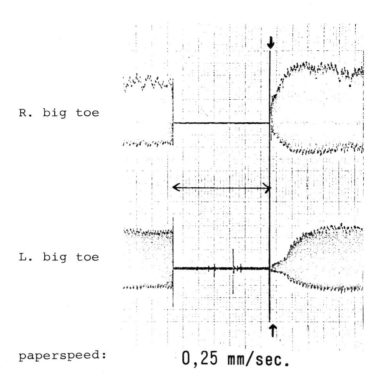

R. big toe

L. big toe

paperspeed: 0,25 mm/sec.

Fig. 5. Photoelectric plethysmogram with arterial occlusion ←——→

D. Doppler bloodpressure measurements

With the transcutaneous Doppler ultrasound echograph ultrasound is sent through the skin above a peripheral artery. The circulating red bloodcells reflect this sound to the receiver (Fig. 6). A cuff is placed around the ankle and inflated above bloodpressure. The Doppler probe is placed above the art. tibialis posterior and the pressure in the cuff is gradually lowered (Fig. 7). At the moment the blood in the artery can pass again the cuff, a sound is heard in the earphone of the echograph, indica-

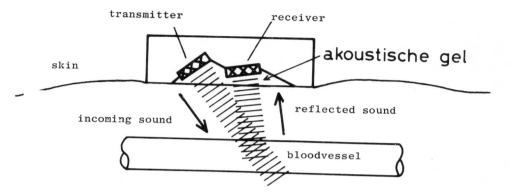

Fig. 6. Probe of Doppler ultrasound apparatus.

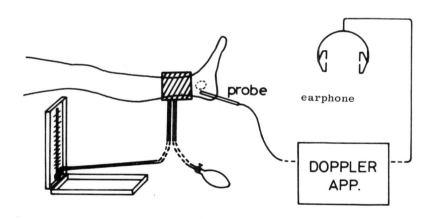

Fig. 7. Doppler bloodpressure measurement ankle.

ting at the bloodpressure manometer the systolic pressure
in the tibial artery. It is also possible to determine in
this way the systolic bloodpressure in the upperleg. The
cuff in this case is placed around the upperleg and for
practical reasons the Doppler probe placed also above the
tibial artery and/or fibular artery. (It is more difficult
to place the detector above the popliteal artery in the
hollow of the knee).

The by this means measured Doppler bloodpressures are
expressed as percentages of the arm bloodpressures. Normally this percentage when measured with the cuff around
the ankle, is 100 % or higher. In case of serious stenosis
and stops in the leg arteries the percentage is < 90 %.
Lower than 50 % is found in patients, already having tro-
phical disturbances of the skin of the legs.

With the cuffs around the upperleg the criteria are
as follows:
> 100 % no serious abnormalities
90-100 % doubtful
< 90 % a) femoral artery with normal pulsations: stenosis
region
b) diminished pulsations of femoral artery: stenosis in iliac artery

It is also possible to measure the Doppler bloodpressure after exercise of the legs. When the pressure after
exercise is lower than in the resting phase, this is also
an indication for a diminished circulation.

These Doppler measurements are a simple screening
method and should be used before deciding to invasive
diagnostic tests as aortography (Hylkema, 1975). The
Doppler bloodpressures of the described patient are shown
in Fig. 1. The percentages in the left upperleg and lower-

leg are very low in the resting state (63 % and 57 %),
diminishing during exercise to respectively 51 % and 54 %.
In the right leg normal percentages are found.

E. More quantitative measurements of the bloodflow in the
legs can be performed with the venous occlusion plethysmography, developed by Whitney (1953) and modified by
Barendsen (1973).

Around the calfs are placed rubber tubes filled with
mercury. Changes in circumference of the calfs cause
changes in the electrical resistance in the mercury tubes,
which can be recorded. Around the upperleg bloodpressure
cuffs are positioned and inflated above venous pressure.
So venous return bloodflow is interrupted, but arterial
flow proceeds normally, causing with every heartbeat aug-
mentation of the volume of the calf, resulting in stretching of the mercury tubes, which can be recorded on the
plethysmograph. In cases of diminished arterial bloodflow
stretching will be less in contradiction to high bloodflow
where stretching will be higher.

In this way it will be possible to measure quantitatively bloodflow in the legs. It is also possible to
measure bloodflow during exercise (patient lying on his
back and moving a pedal with his feet) and after reactive
hypereamia. Barendsen found that maximal bloodflow during
exercise and after stopping for 5 minutes arterial bloodflow by inflating a bloodpressure cuff around the upperleg
above arterial pressure, so causing reactive hyperaemia,
are equal. So it is easier to measure maximal bloodflow
after reactive hyperaemia than during exercise. In the
latter case measurements can be disturbed by the movements
of the legs.

The bloodflow is expressed in ml/100 ml tissue/minute. Normally restflow is between 1 and 5 ml/100 ml/min. Maximal bloodflow after 5 minutes arterial occlusion is normally between 20 and 50 ml/100 ml/minute, ("peakflow"), this peakflow is normally reached in between 10-20 sec ("peakflowtime"). In less than 2 minutes the restflow level is reached again. In cases with diminished bloodflow the peakflow is reached later, is lower and the resting level is reached more slowly. A peakflow of less than 12 ml/100 ml/min is regarded as absolutely pathologic.

Between 12 and 20 ml/100 ml/min is a transistional situation. The venous occlusion plethysmograms of the described patient are shown in Fig. 8.

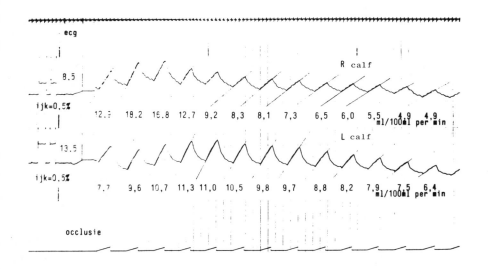

Fig. 8. Semi-continuous venous occlusion plethysmography of the calfs during reactive hyperaemia after arterial occlusion (curves of the described patient).

The maximal flow in the right calf is already reached
in the second measurement after stopping the arterial
occlusion (18.2 ml/100 ml/min), on the left side the maximal flow is lower (11.3 ml/100 ml/min) and only reached
at the fourth measurement. A clear difference between the
two legs is seen. Barendsen automated this volume plethysmograph, so that a number of measurements in the same
patient can be done easily.

These non-invasive methods are important to decide if
there exist pathological conditions in the arteries of the
legs or if the complaints are caused by other diseases,
such as neurological, orthopedic or rheumatic diseases. As
a result of the non-invasive techniques, described above,
it is concluded that the described patient should have a
narrowing of his left iliac artery and therefore aortography should be performed.

Translumbal aortography

Röntgen contrast medium is injected through a needle,
translumbally positioned in the aorta and X-ray pictures
are made of the passing of the contrast medium through the
arteries. The results of the aortogram of the described
patient are shown in Fig. 9.

A stop is seen in the left art. iliaca externa. Collateral vessels are shown, but these are not sufficient to
provide for a normal flow.

Treatment of peripheral atherosclerosis

There are three possible treatments of atherosclerotic
narrowing or stops in peripheral arteries:
1. the best one is the direct surgical treatment. This can

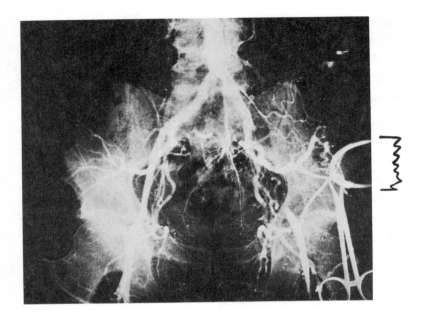

Fig. 9. Aortography of described patient: long stop in
left iliac artery.

be: a desobstruction of the occluded vessel, a venous
by-pass operation (using the saphenous veins as in
coronary artery disease) or in case of obstruction in
the abdominal aorta and the iliac arteries replacement
of the diseased parts by artificial materials (teflon-
grafts a.s.o.).
2. If a direct operation of the vessels is not possible,
in case of multiple lesions or lesions in small vessels,
sometimes lumbar sympathectomy is performed by the surgeon (cutting of the nervus sympathicus).
In our opinion this operation can have good results in
cases with narrowing of smaller arteries in the lower
legs in which case mostly skincomplaints are more im-

portant than muscle complaints. Intermittent claudication is mostly not improved after sympathectomy.

3. Conservative treatment with so called "vasodilating"
   drugs is disappointing. These drugs cause dilatation of
   healthy vessels in other parts of the body and cause
   therefore often a decrease in flow in the diseased already narrowed vessels in the legs (Nieveen, Wouda,
   1975). An example of such a paradoxic reaction is shown
   in Fig. 10. The photoelectric plethysmogram of resp.

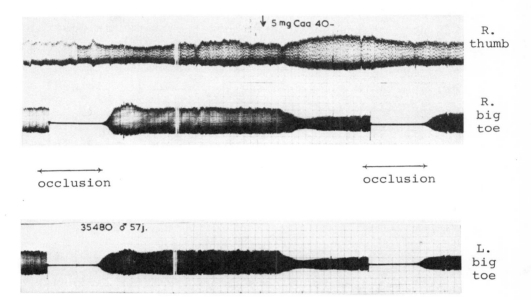

Fig. 10. Photoelectric plethysmogram of R. thumb, R. big
toe and L. big toe before and after i.v. injection of 5 mgr.
Isoxuprine (vasodilating drug). Paradoxic reaction in diseased legs (see text).

right thumb, left and right big toe are shown before
and after injection of a vasodilating drug (5 mgr Ca
40 = Isoxuprine). The amplitudes of the photoelectric
plethysmogram of the diseased legs are decreasing in
contradiction to these of the arms. Elings (1959) has
proven that changing of the amplitude of the photoelectric plethysmogram correlates well with changes in
flow in the same direction. He compared at the same limb
the photoelectric plethysmogram with the venous occlusion plethysmogram.

If none of the above mentioned treatments is possible,
one should try to augment the circulation by training the
patients (walking, eventually on a treadmill, climbing
stairs, cycling a.s.o.), hoping to open more collateral
vessels in this way.

The described patient was operated by the vascular
surgeon. It was possible to desobstruct the occluded vessel. After the operation the patient had no complaints
anymore.

LITERATURE

1. Barendsen, G.J. (1973): Bloodflow in human extremities
   at rest, after arterial occlusion and after exercise.
   Academic Thesis, Groningen.
2. Barendsen, G.J., Berg, Jw. van den (1974): Bloedstroom-
   sterkte in het onderbeen bij patienten met claudicatio-
   klachten. Hartbulletin, 5, 155.
3. Elings, H.S. (1959): Foto-electrische plethysmografie
   met behulp van diffus gereflecteerd licht. Academic
   Thesis, Groningen.

4. Hylkema, B.S. (1975): Tussen polspalpatie en aortografie. Diagnostische betekenis van enkele onbloedige meet-methoden bij ontoereikende bloedvoorziening van de benen. Academic Thesis, Groningen.

5. Nieveen, J. Slikke, L.B. van der, Reichert, W.J. (1956). Photoelectric plethysmography with reflected light. Cardiologia, 29, 160.

6. Nieveen, J. Wouda, A.A. (1975): Vaatverwijdende midde-len. Algemene pharmacotherapie, p. 415, Stafleus Weten-schappelijke Uitgevers Maatschappij, Leiden.

7. Pater, L. de, Berg, Jw. van den, Bueno, A.A. (1962): A very sensitive photoplethysmograph, using scattered light and a photosensitive resistance. Acta Physiol. Pharmacol. Neerl., 10, 378.

8. Ratschow, M. (1959): Angiologie, p. 329, Georg Thieme Verlag, Stuttgart.

9. Whitney, R.J. (1953): The measurement of Volumechanges in human limbs. J. Physiol., 121, 1.

CHAPTER XVIII
THE DOCTOR, THE PATIENT AND HIS HYPERTENSION

Dunning, A.J.

As a clinical problem nothing looks so easy as the treatment of hypertension. The abnormality is present in a large segment of the adult population, the diagnosis can be made by a few careful measurements and treatment can be simple, safe and effective at a very moderate cost to society and as a relatively minor burden both to doctor and patient.

However, hypertension in the population at large is in a majority symptomless and undetected. When sought for it is present in one out of seven people screened, but the consequences of finding it are often minimal. Even when treated the effects are transitory, patient compliance is low and prospective rewards of antihypertensive treatment are rarely harvested.

Although it is known from selected studies on malignant hypertension, carefully controlled investigations in mild hypertension and epidemiology, that antihypertensive treatment may prolong life, avoid strokes, prevent heart failure and even diminish the risks of myocardial infarction our strategy for treatment looks - to say the least - imperfect, often unaccepted and not scientifically based.

Three factors, closely linked together, may be held responsible. The first is our ineptitude in detecting hypertension, the second has to do with the quality of medical care and the third, and most important, with patient acceptance and compliance.

The detection of hypertension

The detection of a symptomless disorder like hypertension depends largely on accidental blood pressure measurement at a check-up, hospital admission or medical examination for jobs or insurance.

Lately screening programs have been advocated to improve the detection rate and some of these programs have been realized in cardiovascular surveys, blood banks, industrial communities and even in shopping centres and county fairs. Doctors and paramedical personnel have been urged to measure blood pressure in every single patient coming to office, clinic or hospital. Even dentists, pharmacists and ophthalmologists are being recruited in case finding, but some critical look at indiscriminate screening is warranted.

If screening is done at a fixed location like a supermarket, only a small section of the target population will be found, in the order of 10 per cent, and any attempt to increase the sample will be costly and time-consuming. The second question is whether in every community such a screening program is warranted, since it is presumed that blood pressure is largely unmeasured in general medical care, a proposition not always proven.

Thus, a screening program in Canada showed that half of the hypertensive persons detected were unaware of their elevated blood pressure, but nearly 80 per cent had their blood pressure measured in the previous two years. Therefore, case finding may detect again a high blood pressure, but demonstrates at the same time that a hypertension found

185

is not a hypertension treated and the patient has to be
linked to a doctor and a system of follow-up and care.

The wisdom of screening programs therefore is debat-
able and at least some preference must be given to educate
practising doctors to measure blood pressure at the first
visit of any patient. Deficiencies in good medical care
are simpler to improve at a smaller cost than the initiation
and upkeep of screening programs.

The treatment of hypertension

Hypertension treatment within current practice need
not be cumbersome or costly and may greatly reduce cardiovascular damage, as the Veterans Administration Studies
have shown. In The Netherlands treatment with a diuretic,
combined with either methyldopa or a β-blocking drug, may
amount to $ 100-200 a year, an investment well worth its
costs.

Since many hypertensive regimes are lifelong, use
multiple drugs in divided dosages which produce side-
effects, treatment may be counterproductive in giving
symptoms while lowering blood pressure.

Some guidelines to treatment warrant discussion and
the first is whether dietary sodium restriction is necessary. Epidemiological surveys have demonstrated a high
incidence of hypertension in countries like Japan and
Korea where salt-intake is excessive, against a nearly
complete absence of hypertension in Amazone Indians, in
certain Pacific islands and New Guinea, where salt-intake
is extremely low. Apart from salt-intake in certain communities, there must be some mechanism or genetic factor
which predisposes for hypertension, since only a part of
the population is affected.

186

Hypertension experts often have said that salt restriction makes life intolerable and is only possible - as
Pickering said - within the religious mind of the fanatic.
However, our craving for salt is a relatively late addict-
ion, probably fostered by salty baby foods and tinned products, where it is used as a conserving salt like our sea-
faring forebears did.

Even moderate salt restriction can produce a diastolic
lowering between 5 and 7 mm Hg in mild hypertension, a
result comparable to that achieved with diurectics. Thus,
it makes no sense to treat the patient with a high dosage
of thiazides and on the other hand make no attempt to reduce his salt-intake to a maximum of six grams salt a day,
which is nearly half the amount consumed in Western societies.

When drug treatment is unavoidable, a choice has to
be made and β-blocking drugs or diuretics are usually the
first. In moderate doses they produce equal effects and a
clear preference if difficult to make. The risks of gout,
carbohydrate intolerance and electrolyte disturbances have
to be weighed against those of bronchospasm, heart failure,
gastro-intestinal disturbances and cold extremities in any
individual patient and often a combination is the most
practical solution.

Since newer β-blocking drugs are effective when taken
once daily, patient compliance may be enhanced and the combination of a long-acting thiazide drug with a new generation of β-blockers is a logical option. The pharmacological choice, however, is only part of the treatment problem, since it is only one aspect of the patient's acceptance of having hypertension and being treated and controlled for it. Thus, the treatment with drugs can never

be isolated from the setting in which this treatment takes place and the opportunity it affords for the patient to comply.

Patient compliance

Any treatment of hypertension has to be judged against its acceptance by the patient. From a healthy individual he or she is degraded by the sphygmomanometer to patient status, compelled to take drugs with potential side-effects and submit himself to lifelong control.

The potential damage of hypertension in old age is not meaningful to a young adult who does not direct his fantasy towards the infirmities of old age. The same failure of imagination makes anti-smoking propaganda rather futile and only those in direct contact with its consequences, chest physicians, surgeons and cardiologists, refrain from smoking as opposed to their psychiatrist brethren. Apart from that, antihypertensive treatment may introduce subtle side-effects like lack of interest, gradual change in sexual behaviour or a general feeling of tiredness, which causes more complaints than the original deviation from normal arterial pressure.

In most studies of drug compliance hypertensive patients default in a quarter, which may be surprisingly low, given human nature. At least these data are superior to those of drug compliance in a far more imaginable disease, pulmonary tuberculosis.

Patient compliance is rarely dependent on a single factor, as social class, age, education or personality. In most cases it is the setting of disease and its treatment which may decide whether the patient is cooperative or not.

Firstly, hypertension causes no typical complaints and headaches, dizziness or tiredness are as common in the population as in hypertensive patients. Although some of them will readily ascribe their subjective complaints to their blood pressure and seek treatment, they will as readily attribute any new complaint to the drugs prescribed for treatment. Therefore the patient should be told from the onset of treatment that he is treated for a chronic symptomless ailment for life in order to avoid hypothetical but severe acute disorders. Many patients and even doctors believe that once treatment has normalized blood pressure it can be omitted, since arterial pressure is normally regulated again. This fallacy is dangerous, since after discontinuation of treatment hypertension returns in 85 % of patients within six months. In those whose blood pressure remains normal the initial hypertension was often minimal or doubtfully established by too few measurements.

The patient has to accept the payment of a lifelong premium for high blood pressure as an insurance against stroke, heart failure or renal damage. Education of the patient, however, is not a short way to better compliance. A Canadian investigation showed a disturbingly high drop-out rate of hypertensive patients just after detection and initial treatment, despite extensive education and facilitating control.

The patient himself performs a critical role and the very poor, the very old and those living in social isolation often fail to keep up appointments. Next to this group there is a curious one that regularly comes for control but fails to take the drugs prescribed. Social class may be important, but it is likely that the quality of treatment and time available for it are more valuable than any other

parameter. There may be no second-class citizens, but
there is second-class medical treatment for those who are
lonely, poor, black, old or any combination of these. American negroes, living in the inner city, have to wait for
hours in overcrowded out-patient departments, are often
treated by changing interns, have no doctor of their own
and cannot pay their prescriptions or have to wait again
at the pharmacy. A poor follow-up system coupled to unem-
ployment and migration may defeat any attempt at treating
a chronic symptomless condition.

Thirdly, the doctor's role can be a critical factor.
Lack of time makes bad doctors and the patient who is
given no opportunity to tell his complaints, whether real
or imaginary, and is hastely given a refill-prescription
after measuring his blood pressure, will certainly drop
out when it becomes convenient. Good medical care requires
some relationship and changing doctors at university clinics therefore perform much worse than a devoted general
practitioner.

There is much discussion and pressure to use paramedical personnel in the control of hypertensive patients
and they surely are as adequate as doctors in maintaining
a follow-up scheme, measuring blood pressure and adapting
drug therapy. It remains to be seen, however, whether they
can replace the contact with a personal physician, inte-
rested not only in arterial pressure but also in the
patient himself.

The nature of drug treatment has great practical value. Academically every patient should have a medication
tailored individually to his needs and blood pressure, but
that may be a clinical pharmacologist's dream. In hypertension the non-pharmacological basis of therapeutics may

190

be equally important and some simple rules are to be obeyed.

The more drugs that are prescribed, the less are taken, especially in the elderly patient who is using sleeping pills, laxatives, sedatives and many others. Since most tablets are small, round and white, a large source of serious mistakes is created. The more often a drug is prescribed, the less it will be taken and many patients simply forget to take a tablet at lunch or during work when prescribed three times a day.

Any drug that can be given once a day, preferably in the morning, like diuretics and many newer β-blocking drugs, like timolol, pindolol and metoprolol or oxprenolol in a matrix form, are therefore to be preferred to others, since they greatly improve compliance.

Lastly, the side-effects may be deciding and in some studies diuretics proved to be far more acceptable than guanethidine, methyldopa or a β-blocking drug, prescribed in divided doses. Apart from that, any complaint will be often ascribed to the particular drug in use, like loss of sleep during diuretic treatment, despite the lack of such an association.

Doctors, until they have been patients themselves, are often unable to imagine the effects of drug treatment in the life of their patients. Therefore they do not enquire about the quality of sexual life under clonidine, reserpine or methyldopa, the vivid dreams, cold extremities or muscle fatigue under β-blocking drugs or the social handicap of using quick-acting diuretics. A good eye for side-effects and their importance in the individual patient is therefore mandatory for successful management.

CHAPTER XIX
TREATMENT OF HYPERLIPIDEMIA

Meinders, A.E.

Arguments for treatment

The lipid hypothesis is the postulate that reducing
the level of plasma cholesterol and triglycerides in an
individual or a population group will lead to a reduction
in the risk of suffering a new event of coronary heart
disease. This hypothesis is founded on the well documented
fact that people with higher plasma cholesterol and triglyceride levels have more and earlier coronary heart disease
than do others with lower levels. There is a continuous correlation between coronary heart disease and plasma cholesterol concentrations which means that no sharp defined cut-off
point exists below which the plasma cholesterol level is no
risk factor anymore. In other words lowering plasma cholesterol levels could be a preventive manipulation for everybody.
Persons to be treated are usually selected by the elevation
of their plasma lipid concentrations. In general one selects
persons who have lipid concentrations above the range in
which 95% of the local population have their plasma lipid
concentrations. However Western European and American populations have higher plasma lipid concentrations than population groups in other parts of the world so that a lower
plasma lipid level than that below which 95% of the plasma
lipid levels of the local population are, might be an errone-
ously high initial concentration for treatment.

It is not only of importance to know the plasma concentrations of low density lipoproteins (LDL, to which most plasma cholesterol is bound) and very low density lipoproteins (VLDL, carrier of endogenous triglycerides), because these concentrations are correlated with coronary heart disease, but also of plasma cholesterol bound to high density lipoproteins (HDL). It is assumed that HDL plays a role as an acceptor for removed cholesterol for instance from the vascular wall. In patients with coronary heart disease (CHD) levels of HDL are lower than normal (up to 35%). The combination of increased LDL and decreased HDL forms a high correlation with coronary heart disease. So HDL seems to protect against atherosclerosis. HDL is proportional to exercise and inversely proportional to obesity, cigarette smoking and VLDL.

Up to the present time four reports (one of which is preliminary) have been published describing the effect of lowering plasma lipid concentrations on coronary heart disease. Diet as well as drug treatment was used for this purpose. During the period of study (usually 5 years) plasma lipid levels decreased 10-20% but no convincing evidence could be produced that this lowering of plasma lipid levels had any beneficial effect on prevention of (primary or secondary) coronary heart disease.

There are several reasons why the negative results of these studies might not be so conclusive that no arguments exist to treat hyperlipidemic patients. A 5-year treatment period might be too short for regression of atheromatous plaques, which have been developed during a whole lifespan. In this respect it is of interest to start treatment at a very young age before atherosclerosis is manifest.

In the studies mentioned so far presumably patients

were studied suffering from type IIA hyperlipoproteinemia whose plasma lipids are least responsive to dietary of drug manipulation and who are most likely to suffer a new event of coronary heart disease within the 5-year study period. Especially in a younger age group during a secondary (coronary heart disease already manifest) study, the number of type IIA hyperlipoproteinemic patients might be considerable (estimated 20% of all survivors of myocardial infarction under age of 60). It seems worthwhile to test if this subgroup differs from the general population in the reaction to changes of plasma lipid concentrations.

One should realize that treatment of hyperlipidemia with diet as well as with drugs is not without side effects. Several of the drugs studied so far had to be removed because of dangerous side effects (dextrothyroxine, estrogens).

Summarizing it can be said that no proof of a beneficial effect (on coronary heart disease) of lowering plasma lipid concentrations is available. As neither the efficacy nor the nontoxicity of lowering plasma lipid levels is proven, it seems premature to make recommendations in this direction to the general population. However the lipid hypothesis has neither been definitely proven wrong so that clinicians shall still treat hyperlipidemia in selected high-risk patients.

Apart from the lipid hypothesis treatment of patients suffering from type IV hyperlipoproteinemia (endogenous hypertriglyceridemia) has the rationale to relieve or avoid complications like eruptive xanthomas, abdominal pain, pancreatitis and hepatosplenomegaly.

The aims for treating the less frequent types I and V hyperlipoproteinemias is to keep the subjects free of bouts of abdominal pain and clear of xanthomas.

194

A rare group of treatable hyperlipidemic patients are
those suffering from type III hyperlipoproteinemia (Broad-
beta-disease, floating beta disease). They form the only
group of patients in whom improvement or regression of arterial lesions especially peripheral arteries is documented
during treatment. Also the xanthomas are readily reversible.

Diet

The uncommon hyperlipoproteinemias

Reduction in dietary fats has been the mainstay of
therapy for familial type I hyperlipoproteinemia. The object is reducing circulating chylomicrons to levels not
associated with symptoms or signs. A diet containing less
than 60 grams of fat per day is well tolerated but sometimes the fat content of the diet must be reduced below
30 grams per day. Medium-chain triglycerides have been used
because they are absorbed into the portal circulation without chylomicron synthesis.

In type III hyperlipoproteinemia dietary control includes two stages. First a low-caloric diet is prescribed
until ideal body weight is achieved followed by a balanced
diet containing 40% calories from carbohydrates, 40% from
fat and 20% from protein. Dietary fats must be low in
cholesterol (less than 300 mg daily) and saturated fatty
acids and high in polyunsaturated fatty acids.

Weight reduction and achieving ideal bodyweight is the
cornerstone of therapy in type V hyperlipoproteinemia.
Thereafter a maintenance diet may be prescribed avoiding
excess of fat and carbohydrates. Dietary fat is restricted
to less than 30% of the total calories.

Type II and IV hyperlipoproteinemia

Weight reduction is stressed particularly in over-weight patients with hypertriglyceridemia. A low carbohydrate diet is seldom required to achieve significant lowering of serum triglycerides in middle-aged, obese, hypertriglyceridemic men, with or without hypercholesterolemia, provided that weight loss is accomplished and sustained and intake of saturated fat and cholesterol is low. Otherwise control of carbohydrate intake (less than 40% of total calories) may be beneficial. No proof exists that withdrawal of simple sugars is more effective than an equivalent decrease of complex carbohydrates.

In type II hyperlipidemic patients diet should be modified so that the total cholesterol intake is reduced (arbitrarily below 300 mg per day), the amount of calories derived from saturated animal fat must be reduced and most of the calories derived from fat has to come from polyunsaturated fatty acids. The rationale for reducing dietary cholesterol comes from studies in which human volunteers showed higher plasma cholesterol concentrations when consuming increasing amounts of cholesterol. This effect of cholesterol is independent of that of dietary fat. Population studies also showed increased plasma cholesterol levels when the intake of cholesterol was higher. The absorption of dietary cholesterol is about 40%, even with very high intake (several grams). However in this latter situation endogenous cholesterol synthesis is decreased and fecal excretion of cholesterol increased. In familial hypercholesterolemia only a minor part of the body stores of cholesterol is derived from dietary cholesterol.

In normal persons as well as in hyperlipidemic patients plasma cholesterol decreases when saturated fatty acids are substituted by polyunsaturated fatty acids. In this context linoleic acid plays the most important role. The mechanism of this plasma cholesterol reducing action of polyunsaturated fatty acids remains to be clarified. The isomeric (cis or trans) configuration does not seem to play a role. An increased fecal excretion of neutral and bile steroids has been found in some studies but not in others and a redistribution of body cholesterol has been postulated. Apart from lowering plasma cholesterol concentrations, linoleic acid might play an important role in decreasing the ill-effects of hyperlipemia, by the increasing prostaglandin synthesis. In their turn these prostaglandins inhibit aggregation and adhesion of circulating thrombocytes, which mechanism may play an important role in arterial thrombosis.

A low cholesterol, low total fat diet with a high content of polyunsaturated fatty acids will result in a decrease of about 20% of plasma cholesterol. One should however be aware of the fact that in patients treated this way more gallbladder disease has been diagnosed.

Drugs

Cholestyramine

Cholestyramine is the chloride salt of a basic anion-exchange resin (trimethylbenzyl-ammonium groups). This resin is orally administered and not absorbed. It exchanges chloride for bile acids in the alimentary tract. The removal of bile acids from the enterohepatic circulation increases the conversion of cholesterol into bile acids and so fecal loss of cholesterol. Unfortunately this process is followed by increased synthesis of cholesterol, which limits the plasma cholesterol lowering effect of the drug.

197

The usual daily dose of cholestyramine is 16 grams or more
divided over at least 2 gifts. Plasma cholesterol levels
may drop about 20-25%. The drug has no effect on HDL
cholesterol and VLDL cholesterol. After stopping the drug
plasma cholesterol and LDL concentrations rise rapidly to
their original levels. Cholestyramine has usually little
or no effect on plasma triglycerides but in some patients
and in normal control subjects elevations during treatment
have been recorded. Homozygous type II^A hyperlipoproteinemic patients do not react favourably as a rule, even if
given doses are as high as 24 grams per day.

Nausea, constipation and, used in high dosages, stea-
torrhea are unpleasant side effects. Very high dosages can
theoretically be accompanied by decreased absorption of
fatsoluable vitamins and hyperchloremic acidosis. Cholestyramine can bind other substances among which concurrent-
ly administered drugs (chlorothiazide,fenylbutazone, anticoagulants, thyroxine and digoxine).

Colestipal and DEAE-Sephadex are more recent bile-
acid sequestrants.

Clofibrate

Clofibrate is the ethylester of p-chlorophenoxy iso-
butyric acid. This drug characteristically reduces the
plasma triglyceride concentration by lowering the levels
of VLDL. In this respect its main use is in treating patients with type IV hyperlipoproteinemia. Very good results
can also be obtained in type III patients. The results
however in type II are questionable whereas the drug is
ineffective in type I and V hyperlipoproteinemia. Several
mechanisms may play a role in the plasmatriglyceride lowering effect. Clofibrate is supposed to be antilipolytic,

followed by a decreased delivery of free fatty acids to the liver. The liver reacts with diminished synthesis of triglycerides. An increased lipoprotein-lipase activity in adipose tissue has been demonstrated, resulting in an increased clearance of plasmatriglycerides. Given in a dose of 2 grams per day plasma triglyceride should drop 20-25%. This lipid lowering effect is manifest within 2-5 days after initiating therapy. Clofibrate has also an effect on plasma cholesterol. One of its mechanisms may be an increased fecal loss of cholesterol and a diminished synthesis of cholesterol with a dminished total body cholesterol pool.

In some patients plasma cholesterol and LDL concentrations rise while triglyceride and VLDL levels fall during treatment with this drug. After discontinuation of the drug a marked rebound of both triglyceride and cholesterol may occur.

Side effects are not frequent. As a major fraction of the drug is bound to plasma albumin, it displaces other drugs and influences thereby their action (coumarine derivatives). Increased serum enzyme activities like GOT, GPT and CPK have been demonstrated. A syndrome of muscle cramps, stiffness and weakness has been ascribed to the drug. Occasionally patients experience nausea,vomiting, loss of libido and painful breasts. During longterm treatment increased gall bladder disease occurs, because of oversaturation of the bile with cholesterol. In the coronary drug project clofibrate treatment was accompanied by an increased incidence of thromboembolism, angina pectoris, intermittent claudication and cardiac arrhythmias.

Nicotinic acid

Nicotinic acid reduces plasma cholesterol as well as plasma triglyceride levels. It does this by lowering plasma LDL and VLDL concentrations. Primarily the drug is supposed to inhibit lipolysis in adipose tissue by decreasing accumulation of cAMP in fat cells. The decreased delivery of free fatty acids to the liver is followed by a decreased triglyceride and VLDL synthesis. The next step is that less VLDL is transformed into LDL and finally plasma cholesterol levels fall. A decreased synthesis and increased catabolism of cholesterol by the liver has also been postulated. The plasma lipid lowering action of the drug is applicable in type II, III, IV and V hyperlipoproteinemia. The usual daily dose is 3 grams. Because of side effects this dose should be reached slowly. The expected fall of plasma triglycerides is 25% and of plasma cholesterol $\pm$ 10%.

Because of the several side effects its usefulness is limited. Of the various side effects the most important are flushes, other cutaneous reactions, gastrointestinal disturbances, glucose intolerance, increased plasma uric acid levels, liver dysfunction and cardiac arrhythmias.

Neomycin

This almost completely nonabsorbable antibiotic is used in type II hyperlipoproteinemia because of its plasma cholesterol lowering effect. The usual daily dose is 0.5-2 grams. Its cholesterol lowering effect is located in the intestinal lumen. Micellar formation is probably reduced with consequently precipitation of bile acid and cholesterol followed by fecal loss of these substances. Because of its antibiotic effect on intestinal bacterial growth also changes in bile acid metabolism and increased fecal loss, occur.

200

The cholesterol lowering effect is $\pm$ 20%.

Diarrhea is its main side effect. One should be careful about hearing loss and renal damage as $\pm$ 3% of the drug is absorbed from the intestinal tract.

Other drugs

Dextrothyroxine and estrogens should not be used because of serious side effects. None of the other advocated drugs have been tested sufficiently to advise their use routinely.

Other ways of treatment

Portocaval shunting has been performed in a small number of homozygous type II^A hyperlipoproteinemia, who were resistant to conventional therapy. Sustained decrease of plasma LDL and cholesterol levels are demonstrated with regression of clinical signs and symptoms, among which apparent improvement of coronary bloodflow. A decreased overall synthesis rate of cholesterol and LDL has been found, the mechanism of which has to be further evaluated.

Plasma exchange using a continuous flow blood-cell separator is followed by a pronounced reduction of plasma LDL and cholesterol in homozygous type II^A hyperlipoproteinemic patients, resistant to conventional therapy. This procedure has to be repeated with about 3-weekly intervals during many months.

Intravenous Hyperalimentation using glucose as the caloric source has been tested in therapy resistant type II^A homozygous hyperlipoproteinemia. Plasma cholesterol falls considerably as does LDL and HDL during therapy and these concentrations remain lowered till 2 weeks after stopping

201

therapy. The mechanism of action of this way of therapy is unknown.

Ileal by-pass lowers cholesterol by preventing reabsorption of bile acids and is therefore a surgical equivalent of a bile acid sequestrant like cholestyramine. The procedure is presumably not more effective than the drug in type II hyperlipoproteinemia.

Literature

1. Ahrens, E.H. (1976): Ann. Int. Med. 85, 87.
2. Ahrens, E.H. (1974): Lancet 2, 449.
3. Bilheimer, D.W. (1977): New Engl. J. Med. 296, 508.
4. Coronary Drug Project (1977): New Engl. J. Med. 296, 1185.
5. Coronary Drug Project (1975): JAMA 231, 360.
6. DeWitt, S., Goodman (1976): in: The year in Metabolism 1975-1976.
7. Editorial Lancet (1977): Lancet 2, 808.
8. Levy, R.I. et al. (1973): Ann. Int. Med. 79, 51.
9. Mann, G.V. (1977): New Engl. J. Med. 297, 644.
10. Miller, N.E. et al. (1977): Lancet 1, 965.
11. Morris, J.N. et al. (1977): BMJ 4, 1307.
12. Rifkind, B.M. (1973): Clin. Endocrinol. Metab. 2, 1.
13. Schade, R.W.B. (1976): Thesis Nijmegen.
14. Starzl, T.E. et al. (1973): Lancet 2, 940.
15. Taylor, K.G. et al. (1977): Lancet 2, 1106.
16. Thomson, G.R. et al. (1975): Lancet 1, 1208.
17. Torsvik, H. et al. (1975): Lancet 1, 601.
18. Yesurun, D. et al. (1976): Am. J. Med. 60, 379.

CHAPTER XX

INDICATIONS AND APPLICATION OF ANTITHROMBOTIC
THERAPY IN ATHEROSCLEROTIC DISEASES

Van Aken, W.G.

INTRODUCTION

In chapter II evidence was presented to support the
hypothesis that thrombotic processes may contribute to
both the development and the sequelae of atherosclerotic
lesions. Therefore it appears relevant to consider now the
effect of so called antithrombotic drugs, on the outcome
of conditions in which atherosclerosis is more or less prominent.

Three classes of drugs have been evaluated for the
management of thrombosis. These are (a) drugs which inhibit fibrin formation (the anticoagulant drugs and defibrinating agents), (b) drugs which prevent platelet adhesion or aggregation (platelet inhibiting drugs) and (c)
drugs which digest fibrin (fibrinolytic agents). On theo-
retical grounds it might be expected that these three groups
of drugs would not be equally effective for prevention and
treatment of venous and arterial thromboembolism. Thus,
anticoagulants and defibrinating agents should be more
effective in venous thromboembolism whereas drugs which
suppress platelet function might be of greater value in
arterial thrombosis. Fibrinolytic substances should be
useful in the treatment of those thrombi of which fibrin
is a major constituent.

With regard to the treatment and prevention of atherosclerotic diseases emphasis has been on the application
of oral anticoagulants and more recently on platelet inhibiting drugs.

ORAL ANTICOAGULANTS

Oral anticoagulants act by interfering with the hepatic synthesis of the Vitamin K-dependent clotting factors,
i.e. factors II, VII, IX and X. There are two types of
vitamin K antagonists, the coumarins and the indanedione
derivatives. The oral anticoagulants are low molecular
weight organic compounds which are rapidly absorbed from
the gastrointestinal tract. They are 90-99 % bound to albumin so that only a small fraction of the amount of the
drug is pharmacologically active at any time. All oral
anticoagulant drugs undergo almost complete metabolic
transformation and are excreted in altered form either in
urine or stool.

These drugs inhibit the effect of vitamin K on a post-
ribosomal step in the hepatic synthesis of clotting factors II, VII, IX and X so that treatment with oral anticoagulants leads to the synthesis of biologically inactive,
but immunologically detectable forms of these clotting
proteins which are called PIVKA's (Protein Induced by
Vitamin K antagonist). These modified proteins lack one of
the -carboxyl groups of the -carboxy-glutamic acid resi-
dues which are responsible for the property of calcium
binding. The lack of calcium binding results in defective
binding of the molecule to phospholipid and hence in impaired conversion of prothrombin to thrombin, which in
turn leads to retardation of fibrin formation.

The antithrombotic effect of these drugs is delayed until the level of normal coagulation factors is reduced till 10 to 20 % of normal. Thus, peak plasma levels of warfarin occur within six hours or oral administration but the maximal hypo-prothrombinemic effect only occurs 36-72 hours after drug administration.

The effect of oral anticoagulants on blood coagulation is commonly measured with either the one stage prothrombin time (PT) or the Thrombotest^R. It should be noted that the results of these clotting tests are dependent on the source and quality of the thromboplastin reagent used. In this respect the Thrombotest appears to be a reliable test.

There is evidence that there is a "therapeutic range" for the anticoagulant effect of these drugs, which is a PT of about twice normal and for the Thrombotest is between 5 and 15 %. When the PT is prolonged more than twice normal or the Thrombotest result is less than 5 % the risk of bleeding is increased.

Traditionally, oral anticoagulant treatment has been started with a loading dose which is followed with progressively smaller doses of the drug until a daily maintenance dose is found which produces the desired therapeutic effect. Either the PT or the Thrombotest should be measured 3 times in the first week and then weekly until the patient's maintenance dose is stable. After this, the effect of treatment can be monitored at two or three week intervals. Several oral anticoagulant preparations with varying pharmacological properties are available. In order to gain optimal personal experience it is useful to select a short and a long acting preparation. The anticoagulant effect of acenocoumarol (Sintrom^R) continues for 1.5 to

2 days after the administration of the drug is discontinued. In contrast the effect of phenprocoumon (Liquamar[R],
Marcoumar[R]) continues for 7 to 14 days. Acenocoumarol is
prefered to be used in clinical situations where rapid
adjustment of the dosage may be necessary. Phenprocoumon
is indicated for the longterm treatment of patients with
an uncomplicated course. Phenidione, an indanedione derivative, is not recommended because its use is associated
with a higher incidence of serious side effects (e.g.
blood dyscrasias) than that of the coumarin compounds.

The major undesirable effect of oral anticoagulant
therapy is bleeding which during well controlled treatment is usually due to surgical or other forms of trauma,
or to a local lesion such as a peptic ulcer of carcinoma.
When the PT or Thrombotest is in the therapeutic range in
medical patients, bleeding is probably not much more frequent than in controls but tends to be more serious. Non-
hemorrhagic side effects with coumarins, notably skin
necrosis, are very rare. If the patient is bleeding during
oral anticoagulant therapy, 10 to 15 mg vitamin K_1 should
be given intravenously. Vitamin K_1 must not be given faster
than 5 mg per minute because more rapid injection may produce adverse reactions like tachycardia, hypotension,
dyspnoe and flushing. In most patients intravenous vitamin
K_1 has a demonstrable effect on the PT (or Thrombotest)
within 3 to 4 hours of injection. When short acting preparations (e.g. coumarin) are used, safe levels of clotting
factors are reached within 6 to 8 hours and oral treatment with 2.5 to 10 mg vitamin K_1 for 2 days is usually
sufficient. In case the patient is, however, treated with
long-acting oral anticoagulants (e.g. Marcoumar) repeated
control of the PT is necessary and vitamin K_1 should be ad-

ministered over a longer period.

Replacement therapy with a concentrate of factors II, VII, IX and X is indicated when immediate correction of the drug induced coagulation defect is required, such as in patients with suspected cerebral hemorrhage and respiratory tract bleeding.

A number of factors affect the anticoagulant response of patients to oral anticoagulant drugs. The most important is the action of other drugs. These drugs may reduce the absorption of vitamin K, alter coumarin absorption, alter the rate of inactivation of coumarins by hepatic enzyme systems and most important reduce binding of anticoagulants to albumin and so increase the concentration of pharmacologically active drug. This last effect is the most common mechanism of an increased anticoagulant effect and occurs by the administration of e.g. phenylbutazone, aspirin, chloral hydrate and long-acting sulfonamides. Barbiturates increase the rate of hepatic inactivation of enzyme induction of coumarins which results in a more rapid clearance of the anticoagulant and hence in a lessened anticoagulant effect. The list of drugs which interfere with oral anticoagulant treatment is too long to remember, but it should be kept in mind that changes of concomitant drug therapy should be kept to the minimum. If a change must be made, the PT or Thrombotest should be monitored frequently for several weeks after the new drug is introduced or after the drug has been withdrawn.

In addition increased sensitivity of oral anticoagulants is seen in patients with reduced liver function, vitamin K deficiency, congestive heart failure, diarrhea and hypermetabolic states (e.g. fever, thyreotoxicosis).

Oral anticoagulants are contraindicated in patients with blood dyscrasias, ulceractive lesions of the gastro-intestinal tract, recent surgery or trauma of the central nervous system, chronic alcoholism, malignant hypertension, serious liver disease and during the first and last trimester of pregnancy.

Clinical evaluation of oral anticoagulant therapy

Since the discovery of the first coumarin derivative by Link in 1943 a large number of clinical trials have been performed to evaluate the use of anticoagulants in patients with acute myocardial infarction. In addition the efficacy of anticoagulant therapy has been investigated in cerebro vascular disease, prosthetic heart valves, mitral valvular disease, and atrial fibrillation, peripheral vascular disease and of course venous thromboembolism. The application of oral anticoagulants in these conditions is based on the possible prevention of fibrin formation which causes deep venous thrombosis, pulmonary embolism and intracardiac mural thrombi. At the time that the value of oral anticoagulant therapy was started to be studied, it was postulated by a number of investigators that thrombus formation in the coronary and cerebral circulation caused myocardial and cerebral infarction. Anticoagulant therapy was expected to prevent the formation and extension of these thrombi.

Coronary artery disease

Most studies reveal a reduction of thromboembolic phenomena in patients with acute myocardial infarction who are taking oral anticoagulants. A significant reduction in deep venous thrombosis as detected by I^{125}-fibrinogen legscanning, was noticed in patients with acute myocardial infarction while on anticoagulant therapy with coumarin derivatives (Nicolaides et al., 1971). Systemic embolism, apparently derived from intracardiac mural thrombi, is also diminished by these drugs (Ebert, 1969). It has also been demonstrated that these favourable results are related to the intensity of anticoagulation. There is, however, still no unanimity about the efficacy of oral anticoagulants in preventing recurrent myocardial infarction and death from myocardial infarction. Originally the results of a large clinical trial reported by Wright et al. (1948) gave evidence that the use of anticoagulants caused a sharp reduction in both thromboembolism and mortality from myocardial infarction. Following this report, the use of anticoagulants became a part of the accepted treatment of acute myocardial infarction. Subsequently, several large clinical trials (Hilden et al., 1961; Working Party on Anticoagulant Therapy in Coronary Thrombosis, 1969; Veterans Administration Cooperative Clinical Trial, 1973) have failed to demonstrate a significant decrease in mortality resulting from the use of anticoagulants and have cast doubt on the value of this therapy. On the other hand some investigators claim that anticoagulants significantly reduce recurrent myocardial infarction and mortality provided that the intensity of hypocoagulability is sufficient (Thrombotest values of 5-12 %) (Loeliger et al., 1967; Meuwissen et al., 1969).

These controversial results oblige a critical analysis before (long-term) anticoagulant therapy can be recommended for large groups of patients with myocardial infarction. The following data appear to be the most important for such considerations:

1. The statistical data in the majority of studies on anticoagulant treatment were obtained without adequate attention to the fundamental principles for the design of clinical investigations. Gifford and Feinstein (1969) established eight methodologic standards that are necessary to ensure comparability of groups of patients in a clinical trial. Using these criteria in a large number of articles on anticoagulant therapy of myocardial infarction, they found that none satisfied all standards and that only four studies satisfied more than 4 of the 8 criteria. Of particular significance was the finding that anticoagulant therapy appeared to be superior to no therapy relatively more often when standards were not met than when they were. Claims of success with coumarin treatment in patients with impending myocardial infarction have also been made, but again the control groups of these studies were not randomly selected. Consequently the value of anticoagulant treatment in these patients is not established.

2. In evaluating long-term therapy it is to be emphasized that survival is the yardstick by which therapeutic results must be measured. In patients with transmural myocardial infarction the death rate during the first 3 months after admission has been reported to be 21 % as compared to 6.6 % during the following 6 months and 5.6 % during the second year after the infarction occurred (Master and Lassen, 1969). Thereafter the mortality in these patients decreased to about 2 % which is hardly different from the mortality in the same age group of the general population. Clinical trials which showed a beneficial effect of oral anticoagulants bear upon relatively

small numbers of patients which started anticoagulant therapy 4 to 12 months following myocardial infarction, i.e. at a time that a favourable effect would be expected to become apparent only when large groups were studied.

3. How frequent is thrombusformation in the coronary arteries the cause of acute myocardial infarction? Roberts and Baju (1972) have established that the incidence of thrombi in the coronary arteries of patients with fatal myocardial infarction was 39 %. Only 8 %, however, of the coronary arteries from patients dying within 6 hours after their acute infarction showed thrombi and in those with fatal subendocardial infarction, thrombi were nearly always absent. In contrast, 50 % of patients dying later than 6 hours after the acute transmural infarction were found to have one or more occluding thrombi. Among these patients the major determinants of the cause of coronary artery thrombosis appeared to be the presence of cardiac shock and congestive heart failure. Thus, it may be questioned if the occluding thrombus in these cases was merely the result rather than the cause of myocardial infarction. Additional evidence to support this was supplied by the observation of radioactivity at necropsy in coronary arterial thrombi in patients that had been given ^{125}I fibrinogen some time after the onset of myocardial infarction (Erhardt et al., 1973).

Although theoretic considerations and experience from past studies would not support further prospective studies on the treatment of acute myocardial infarction with oral anticoagulants, a large scale trial in patients over the age of 60 years, who presented with myocardial infarction, is now in progress in The Netherlands.

Early in this century it was already suggested that
occlusive vascular disease of the carotid arteries was
causally related to stroke and that one of the symptoms of
cerebral disease arising from this relationship was cerebral intermittent claudication. The term transient ischemic
attack (TIA) was born to denote episodes of temporary and
focal cerebral dysfunction of vascular origin, commonly
lasting 2 to 15 minutes and occasionally as long as 24
hours. Of this group of patients, approximately one third
will have irreversible cerebral infarction, one third will
have recurrent attacks and the remainder will have no
further attacks during a follow-up period of 5 years. Although it is not possible to predict whether the patient
describing a typical attack of TIA will have a stroke, it
may be estimated that there is about a 7 % per year risk
of a stroke in a patient who presents with multiple TIA's
and that the risk is greatest in the first few months
after the presenting attack. Investigators disagree about
the pathophysiology of TIA's, implicating hemodynamic factors or emboli of platelets-fibrin and atheromatous
material, usually of carotid origin but sometimes from the
heart. Some may be caused by repeated transient thrombotic
occlusion of the internal carotid artery. Not surprisingly
then, the outcome of several clinical studies regarding
anticoagulant therapy has varied. The aim of anticoagulant
therapy in TIA is to reduce the frequency of attacks and
more important to prevent major stroke and death. Twelve
anticoagulation studies on patients with TIA's have appeared
in the past two decades. As in the majority of studies on
coronary artery disease, the statistical data were obtained
without adequate attention to the fundamental principles

212

for the design of clinical trials. Of the 12 studies, three did not state whether anticoagulants affected the frequency of TIA's, five found fewer attacks among treated patients, three found little or no difference and one observed more attacks while the patients were on anticoagulant therapy (Brust, 1977). It is at present not possible to present firm evidence that oral anticoagulants are effective in the prophylaxis of stroke and death in this patient group. With all studies to date lacking either randomized controls or statistical significance it remains unproven that anticoagulants may be of value in the treatment of TIA.

Prosthetic heart values

Thromboembolism is one of the most frequent serious complications in patients with prosthetic valves. Clinically evident thromboembolism has been reported in 44 % of cases where prophylactic anticoagulation was not employed whereas in patients receiving prophylactic anticoagulation the incidence was reduced to 19 % (Friedly et al., 1971; Gadboys et al., 1967). The incidence varies widely with different valves and control of anticoagulant therapy.

Mitral valvular disease and atrial fibrillation

The triad of rheumatic heart disease, mitral valve stenosis and atrial fibrillation has long been associated with emboli to various organs. Mainly on the basis of the observations of Wright and McDevitt (1954) oral anticoagulants are administered often, starting treatment after the first embolic event. The anticoagulant therapy must be

213

continued indefinitely in these patients unless sinus
rythm is restored (Carter, 1963).

Peripheral arterial disease

No conclusive data are available to allow definite
recommendations on the use of oral anticoagulants in patients with peripheral vascular disease. Using repeated
arteriography Tillgren et al. (1963) studied 74 patients
with intermittent claudication over three years. Some of
these patients were treated with anticoagulants, but
selection criteria are not described. This is important as
the natural course of obliterative arterial disease may
vary considerably in different patients. Patients with oral
anticoagulant therapy developed less often total occlusion
than untreated patients. Existing total occlusions showed
less tendency to grow in the anticoagulant group than in
the control group. In case intermittent claudication is a
consequence of systemic embolism during atrial fibrillation, oral anticoagulant therapy appears to be indicated.

PLATELET INHIBITING DRUGS

The potential of platelet inhibiting drugs rests in
their ability to interfere with platelet reactions which
are associated with thrombosis. Platelets contribute to
thrombosis by adhering to surfaces, by forming aggregates,
by releasing proteolytic enzymes and other factors which
produce endothelial injury and increase vessel permeability. In addition platelets release a mitogenic factor which
induces smooth muscle cell migration into the intima and
the proliferation of these cells which causes intima
thickening. Although the effects of a wide variery of drugs

214

on platelet function have been examined in vitro and in experimental animals, only relatively few have been studied in man in terms of their potential value in the management of arterial thrombosis. In the selection of drugs for clinical use, it would be valuable to have laboratory methods to evaluate the antithrombotic efficacy and dosage. No such tests are currently available and it is not known which aspect of platelet function requires suppresion to achieve such antithrombotic effects. Therefore the assessment of platelet inhibiting drugs depends on the results of clinical trials using prevention of thrombosis-related events as endproducts. In this review only those drugs which in clinical trials have been tested and eventually may show to have some value in man, will be discussed.

Mode of action of the platelet-inhibiting drugs tested in clinical trials

During the last few years a large number of articles have been published about the pharmacological modification of platelet functions. In this review the objective has been to be selective rather than to catalogue. Several detailed reviews of this subject have been published (Weiss, 1975, 1976; Packham and Mustard, 1977; Verstraete, 1976; Genton et al., 1975).

Aspirin

Aspirin (acetylsalicylic acid) like indomethacin and phenylbutazone inhibits collagen induced platelet aggregation and the second phase of aggregation induced by ADP and epinephrine.

One, and perhaps the most important, mechanism of action of aspirin has recently been clarified. Aspirin in

a dosage of 300 mg inhibits the cyclo-oxygenase of platelets and thus blocks the conversion of arachidonic acid to
cyclic endoperoxides (Prostaglandin G_2 and H_2) which give
rise to thrombaxane A_2 (see scheme 1); all these products
can induce the platelet release reaction and aggregation.
There is no good evidence that aspirin can inhibit platelet adhesion to collagen and to subendothelial structures.
The smooth muscle cell proliferation found with vascular
injury does not appear to be inhibited by aspirin.

SCHEME 1 - Inhibition of platelet aggregation by aspirin

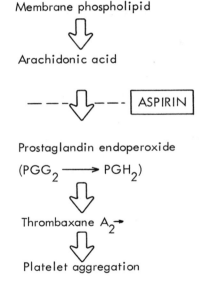

Aspirin is cleared rapidly from the circulation but
the in vitro effects on platelet function are present for
up to 5 days. In addition a single dose of aspirin has
been shown to prolong the bleeding time for almost 5 days

in normal volunteers. This prolonged action is consistent with the view that aspirin has an irreversible effect on all platelets that are circulating at the time of its admission.

Unlike some other platelet inhibiting drugs, aspirin does not prolong the reduced platelet survival seen in a number of vascular diseases.

The commonly used dose of aspirin as an antithrombotic drug is 300 mg given 3 to 4 times per day; theoretically, however, 300 mg per day might be sufficient.

Sulphinpyrazone

Sulphinpyrazone is a uricosuric agent that inhibits the platelet release reaction with collagen and epinephrine but does not prolong the bleeding time. It was recently demonstrated that sulphinpyrazone is a competitive inhibitor of platelet prostaglandin synthesis. Sulphinpyrazone has also been shown to inhibit the adhesion of platelets to subendothelium.

The drug has a plasma half-life of about 2 hours. There is some evidence from experimental animals that the effect of sulphinpyrazone on platelet function may last long after the drug has been cleared which suggests that the effect of sulphinpyrazone might be produced by a metabolite of the drug.

The proliferation of smooth muscle cells which occurs with vascular injury is inhibited by sulphinpyrazone. It has also been shown to prolong the reduced platelet survival time seen in patients with prosthetic heart valves, rheumatic valve disease, gout and coronary artery disease.

The sulphinpyrazone dose used in clinical trials to assess its potential antithrombotic effect is 600 to 800 mg/day.

Dipyridamole

Dipyridamole, initially introduced as a vasodilator, inhibits platelet-aggregation and the platelet release reaction induced by most aggregating agents. However, these effects cannot be demonstrated ex-vivo when dipyridamole is used in pharmacological doses in man and the drug does not prolong the bleeding time. Although the mode of action is not entirely understood, one of the effects of dipyridamole is the inhibition of platelet phosphodiesterase which results in an increase of cyclic AMP levels within the platelets.

In addition, dipyridamole inhibits platelet adhesion to collagen and to subendothelial structures. Dipyridamole has been shown to prevent the shortening of platelet survival that occurs with the injury to the endothelium caused by experimental homocystinemia. This effect appears to be associated with inhibition of smooth muscle cell proliferation in response to endothelial injury. Thus, in experimental animals homocystine-induced atherosclerosis is reduced by the administration of dipyridamole. Also in man this drug prolongs the reduced platelet survival which occurs in a number of thrombovascular conditions.

The dose of dipyridamole used in patients with prosthetic heart valves is 400 mg/day. In some reports this dose has caused side effects (headache, nausea and vomiting) in up to 25 % of patients.

Clofibrate

This hypolipidemic agent inhibits collagen-induced

218

platelet aggregation and the second phase of ADP induced aggregation. It also appears to reduce platelet adhesiveness to glass and latex particles in vitro. Further support for its action as a platelet inhibiting drug is provided by studies which demonstrate that the drug prolongs reduced platelet survival in some patients with coronary artery disease.

Clofibrate has been found to decrease the sensitivity of platelets to aggregating agents in patients with familial hyperbetalipoproteinemia. The mechanism of platelet hypersensitivity in this type II disorder is unknown. Platelets may incorporate total low-density lipoproteins or components into their membranes and thus alter their surface characteristics. The administration of clofibrate could possibly indirectly normalize platelet function. There is as yet no firm evidence for a direct platelet inhibiting effect of clofibrate. It is neither known if clofibrate does prolong the reduced platelet survival in a number of vascular diseases nor is it clear if this drug affects smooth muscle cell proliferation.

The recommended dose of clofibrate as a hypolipidemic drug is 1.5 to 2.0 gr/day; the same dose was used in clinical trials to assess its antithrombotic effect.

Propranolol

Propranolol inhibits the second phase of ADP induced platelet aggregation and platelet adherence to collagen but the mechanism of its action is not clear. Since propranolol displaces calcium from membrane sites it may exert its inhibitory effects on platelets by affecting the calcium concentration in the cytosol.

Interestingly the administration of propranolol to patients with angina pectoris has been shown to reduce the increased sensitivity to ADP induced platelet aggretion and to improve exercise tolerance. This observation raised the question whether reversal of platelet sensitivity to ADP after propranolol administration was a consequence of the improved exercise tolerance. At present data about a possible effect of propranolol on platelet survival and on smooth muscle cell proliferation are lacking. Although a number of clinical trials with propranolol in patients with coronary artery disease have been performed, the contribution of platelets was not explicitly investigated.

Combination of drugs

Since a number of mechanisms are involved in the platelet interactions that result in thrombus formation, and different drugs affect different mechanisms, the possibility exists that combinations of drugs could have greater effects than drugs used singly. There is some evidence that the combination of oral anticoagulants with platelet inhibiting drugs may be beneficial in patients with prosthetic heart valves. Dipyridamole and aspirin have been found to potentiate each other's inhibitory effects on thrombosis involving small vessels. Finally, it has been suggested that a smaller dose (100 to 200 mg/day) of dipyridamole can be used if this drug is combined with aspirin because this combination normalizes the reduced platelet survival in a number of thromboembolic disorders to the same extent as dipyridamole alone.

Clinical evaluation of platelet inhibiting drugs

It would appear that the most useful clinical models for investigating the effects of platelet inhibiting drugs are: transient ischemic attacks (TIA's) and stroke, coronary artery disease, embolization from prosthetic heart valves, and arterial thrombosis. The application of these agents in these situations is based on the possible prevention of platelet thrombus formation and on the embolization of this thrombus. Controlled clinical trials in this area have only recently been started and a number of these studies is still in progress.

Transient cerebral ischemic attacks

Observations of the stenotic lesions at the origin of the internal carotid arteries strongly suggest that it is not the atherosclerotic lesion per se but superimposed thrombotic changes beginning with platelet aggregation, which provide the pathogenic basis for most TIA's.

Four platelet inhibiting drugs have been evaluated in cerebrovascular disease. These studies have been limited to four randomized prospective trials, with placebo-treated concurrent controls, one retrospective study and a number of case reports.

Acheson et al. (1969) evaluated the effect of dipyridamole in patients with TIA or stroke. There was no evidence of a reduction in the frequency of TIA's, stroke or death. However, the number of patients was small, the length of the study relatively short and the incidence of endpoints (stroke or death) was low.

The effect of clofibrate was studied in patients with hypercholesterolemia and TIA or stroke (Acheson and Hutchinson, 1972). No difference in the endpoints was found although a reduction in cholesterol was noted in the treated group.

A retrospective study in patients with TIA to evaluate the effect of aspirin did not show a difference in cerebral infarction and death between the treated and the control group but it was suggested that there was a reduction in the frequency of TIA's in the patients who had been taking aspirin (Dyken et al., 1973). This retrospective study is, however, difficult to interpret since the basis for patient selection was not specified and differences in the follow-up period existed.

Recently a large cooperative controlled study evaluating the effect of aspirin in patients with TIA has been completed (Fields et al., 1977). Analysis of the first six months of follow-up revealed a significant difference in favour of aspirin when death, cerebral or retinal infarction and the occurrence of TIA's were grouped and considered together as endpoints. Significance in favour of aspirin treatment was mainly revealed in patients with a history of multiple TIA's and was most evident in those patients having carotid lesions appropriate to the TIA symptoms. It cannot be inferred from this study that aspirin prevents stroke because there was no statistically significant difference between the aspirin and the placebo treatment when endpoints were restricted to death and cerebral infarction.

A multicentre trial in Canada comparing the effects of aspirin, sulphinpyrazone, aspirin combined with sulphinpyrazone and placebo in patients with TIA has been in progress for five years. Follow-up for the study was terminated in June 1977 but the results are not yet available.[*]

A double blind crossover study in which each of 20

[*] See Addendum

patients with amaurosis fugax, a variant of TIA characterized by accompanying periods of loss of vision, received either sulphinpyrazone or placebo, revealed a significant reduction in episodes of TIA while the patients
were on sulphinpyrazone (Evans, 1972). This study is,
however, limited in that it did not include the more important endpoints of death and stroke. Case reports by
Harrison et al. (1971) and Mundal et al. (1972) also demonstrated that aspirin reduced the number of attacks of
transient blindness.

In conclusion none of these reports have established
the efficacy of platelet inhibiting drugs in terms of
stroke and death but there is evidence that aspirin may
prevent TIA's.

Coronary artery disease

Indirect evidence that platelet inhibiting drugs
might protect against myocardial infarction is already
available from a necropsy study by Cobb et al. (1953). It
was established that only 4 % of a series of patients with
chronic rheumatoid arthritis and taking ant-inflammatory
drugs, had died from myocardial infarction, compared with
31 % of myocardial infarction deaths in the general population.

Three platelet inhibiting drugs have been evaluated
in five prospective randomized secondary prevention studies.

Two multicenter trials evaluated clofibrate in patients who had symptoms of angina pectoris and or evidence
of myocardial infarction (Group of Physicians of the New
Castle upon Tyne Region, 1971; Research Committee of the
Scottish Society of Physicians, 1971). In the New Castle
trial there was a significant reduction in sudden death

and in all deaths in the group of patients receiving clofibrate. In the Scottish trial clofibrate did not reduce
the overall death rate; however, patients with angina
showed a significant reduction both in sudden deaths and
in total mortality when receiving clofibrate. A disquieting feature of these studies was the finding that the
death rate for patients admitted with myocardial infarction
only, was higher for clofibrate than for placebo. Both
studies have been criticized for some aspects of study
design, methodology and analysis (Feinstein, 1972). Convincing evidence for a lack of effect of clofibrate in
patients with myocardial infarction was provided by the
Coronary Drug Project Research Group (1975). No benefit
of clofibrate was found in total mortality and cause specific mortality either for the whole group or for identified subgroups. This study does not exclude the possibility that clofibrate might be effective in patients with
angina.

An international study is currently undertaken to
determine whether the incidence of ischemic heart disease
can be reduced by lowering increased cholesterol levels in
healthy men by the use of clofibrate (Heady, 1973).

A controlled trial of dipyridamole, 400 mg daily, in
103 patients with acute myocardial infarction of less than
two weeks' standing, showed no difference in the number of
complications or deaths during the 28 days observation
period, in either the control or treated group (Gent et al.,
1968). A large number of studies have been performed in
which the anti-anginal effect of dipyridamole was evaluated. However, most of these trials were uncontrolled and
the results regarding angina were inconclusive.

A large-scale multicenter trial, called the Persantin-

Aspirin Re-Infarction Study (PARIS) has been in progress since 1975. In this study 2000 patients who had a myocardial infarction not more than 3 years previously, will receive either a placebo, 1 g of aspirin or 1 g of aspirin combined with 225 mg dipyridamole daily. The follow-up period will be 2 years and the endpoints are recurrent myocardial infarction and death.

Several studies of the role of aspirin in the prevention of myocardial infarction, particularly the secondary prevention, have been performed. Elwood et al. (1974) reported a multicenter, randomized double blind trial of aspirin, in a dose of 300 mg/day, in men with a recent, less than 10 months old, myocardial infarction. During a follow-up for 30 months, a life table analysis showed a trend in reduction of mortality but the difference was not statistically significant. It is of interest that for men whose infarction was of less than 6 weeks duration at entry to the study, the overall mortality was 7.8 % in the aspirin group as compared to 13.2 % in the placebo group which is a statistically significant difference. The Boston Collaborative Drug Surveillance Group (1972) compared the frequency of aspirin ingestion in patients with acute myocardial infarction with those with other diagnoses. The incidence of aspirin ingestion was significantly lower in the myocardial infarction group, being 0.9 % as compared with 4.9 % in the other group. The interpretation of these retrospective studies is, however, always hampered by the possibility of selection bias. Two multicenter trials of aspirin in the secondary prevention of myocardial infarction, apart from the PARIS, are now in progress. The Medical Research Council of Great Britain has started a study in which patients with prior myocardial infarction will be randomized in either placebo or aspirin groups within a few days after infarction. Similarly in the Aspirin Myocardial Infarction Study (AMIS) patients with a myocardial infarction occuring 2 months to 3 years previously are allocated to 1 gr aspirin daily of placebo. In both studies the endpoints of interest are death and the AMIS also recurrent myocardial infarction.

The effect of sulphinpyrazone on cardiac mortality in patients with a recent myocardial infarction is studied at present by a combined American-Canadian group. The first preliminary report of this study (The Anturane Reinfarction Trial Research Group, 1978), at an average follow-up period of 8.4 months, indicate a beneficial effect of sulphinpyrazone in reducing total mortality, cardiac mortality and sudden cardiac death in these patients. The annual sudden-cardiac death rate was 6.3 % for the placebo and 2.7 % for the sulphinpyrazone group, representing a 57.2 % reduction in sudden-cardiac death rate. However, there was only a small reduction in reinfarction rate. This study will be continued till all patients have been followed for a minimum of one year.

The effect of oral anticoagulants, aspirin and placebo on aortocoronary vein graft patency rates was recently reported (McEnany et al., 1976). At 6 to 40 months post-operatively 84 % of the grafts were patent in the patients receiving oral anticoagulants, compared to 80 % in the aspirin group and 72 % in the placebo group. Only the difference between oral anticoagulants and placebo was significant.

In summary, a conclusive effect of platelet inhibiting drugs on the secondary prevention of myocardial infarction has up to now not been shown although sulphinpyrazone appears to reduce cardiac mortality, and more specifically sudden cardiac death rate, in this group of patients. There remains the possibility that platelet inhibiting drugs are of major value in the primary prevention of myocardial infarction or that this form of secondary prevention should be started immediately after myocardial infarction in order to be effective. It remains to be evaluated whether patients considered to be with impending infarction will benefit from this treatment.

Prosthetic heart valves

Several authors have reported that in patients with prosthetic heart valves a relationship exists between shortened platelet survival and thromboembolic complications despite adequate anticoagulation (Harker and Slichter, 1972; Weily et al., 1974). The same authors have shown that both dipyridamole and sulphinpyrazone, but not aspirin, increase the shortened platelet survival towards normal in these patients. Two randomized prospective studies reported data which indicate that the addition of either dipyridamole or aspirin to coumarin is more effective than oral anticoagulants alone in preventing thromboembolic complications in this condition. Sullivan et al. (1971) found that during the one year of observation emboli developed in 14 % of patients with oral anticoagulant therapy as compared to 1.3 % in the group that received in addition 400 mg dipyridamole daily. Recently Dale (1977) performed a double blind study of the effects of 1 gr aspirin combined with oral anticoagulants compared with oral anticoagulants alone in patients with aortic ball valve prosthesis. The incidence of embolism was significantly lower in the combined aspirin-oral anticoagulant group than in the anticoagulant group alone. After the study was completed the patients were treated with aspirin only but this was followed by a high incidence of systemic embolism.

In conclusion the combination of oral anticoagulants with dipyridamole or aspirin is more effective in reducing systemic embolism from prosthetic heart valves than oral anticoagulants alone. In view of the fact that aspirin induces a hemostatic defect and interferes with oral anticoagulants, dipyridamole should be selected for this combined treatment.

Peripheral arterial disease

Only a few studies have been reported on the use of treatment with platelet inhibiting drugs in these disorders. Two prospective studies evaluating aspirin have been reported in patients undergoing arterial catheterization. Both failed to demonstrate a beneficial effect of the platelet inhibiting drug on reduced blood flow to the extremity (Hynes et al., 1973; Freed et al., 1974).

Blakely and Gent (1975) have studied the effect of either sulphinpyrazone or placebo in 169 patients undergoing peripheral vascular surgery for peripheral vascular disease. Drug efficacy was assessed using as endpoints occlusion at the operative site, occlusion in the same leg and all peripheral vascular events. There was no statistically significant difference with respect to any of these endpoints.

Several investigators have made observations with intermittent arterial ischemia of the extremities. Vreeken and van Aken (1971) described a patient with recurrent painful and cyanotic toes who had a moderately elevated platelet count and so-called in vitro spontaneous platelet aggregation. Treatment with dipyridamole was without effect but aspirin treatment, 300 mg daily, was associated with prolonged control of symptoms and concurrent disappearance of spontaneous platelet aggregation. Subsequently, several other authors have made similar observations in patients with thrombocytosis (Bierme et al., 1972; Preston et al., 1974; Mundall et al., 1972).

PERSONAL RECOMMENDATIONS

The following recommendations represent the author's personal opinion about antithrombotic therapy.

In patients with acute myocardial infarction oral anticoagulants are indicated to prevent venous thromboembolism and systemic embolism derived from intracardiac mural thrombosis. The decision for oral anticoagulant treatment should only be taken considering advantages and potential problems related to this form of treatment. Accurate control of treatment and a high degree of patient compliance are obligatory. In addition the interference of other drugs with anticoagulant treatment may cause serious side effects (e.g. hemorrhage). The duration of anticoagulant treatment in acute myocardial infarction is a matter of controverse. We would advocate that this form of prevention is not indicated for more than 2 years after the onset of infarction and certainly not life-long.

Sulphinpyrazone appears to be effective in reducing cardiac deaths during the first year after myocardial infarction. Until the Anturane Reinfarction Trial is completed this platelet function inhibiting drug may be recommended in patients with a recent myocardial infarction.

Patients who present with symptoms of impending myocardial infarction (unstable angina) are unlikely to benefit from oral anticoagulants. Until the results of clinical trials of platelet inhibiting drugs are published, it would appear that sulphinpyrazone and aspirin may protect a number of these patients against infarction and/or sudden death. In view of its lack of side-effects sulphinpyrazone may be selected over aspirin. How long sulphinpyrazone should be administered is unknown. As long as the stimulus for platelet aggregation, i.e. the athero-sclerotic lesion, is present, inhibition of platelet functions may appear to be advantageous.

Long-term treatment with oral anticoagulants is indicated in patients with prosthetic heart valves as well as in mitral valve stenosis and atrial fibrillation. When despite adequate anticoagulation recurrent systemic embolism occurs, dipyridamole should be added. Also in patients with aortocoronary vein grafts long-term oral anticoagulant treatment appears to be indicated.

In patients with TIA's aspirin treatment may be indicated to prevent recurrent attacks and possibly also complete stroke.

There is no evidence that either oral anticoagulant therapy or platelet inhibiting drugs are indicated in patients with peripheral arterial disease. However, in case intermittent claudication is a consequence of systemic embolism, oral anticoagulant therapy is indicated. Lastly in patients with so-called spontaneous platelet aggregation and peripheral ischemia aspirin appears to be of benefit.

REFERENCES

1. Acheson, J., Danta, G., Hutchinson, E.C. Controlled trial of dipyridamole in cerebral vascular disease. Brit. Med. J., 1, 614, 1969.

2. Acheson, J., Hutchinson, E.C. Controlled trial of dipyridamole in cerebral vascular disease. Atherosclerosis, 15, 177, 1969.

3. Anturane Reinfarction Trial Research Group: Sulfinpyrazone in the Prevention of Cardiac Death after Myocardial Infarction. New Engl. J. Med., 298, 289, 1978.

4. Biermé, T., Boneu, R., Guiraud, B., Pris, J. Aspirin and recurrent painful toes and fingers in thrombocythaemia. Lancet, 1, 432, 1972.

5. Blakely, I.A., Gent, M. Platelets, drugs and longevity in a geriatric population, 284 In: Hirsh, Cade, Gallus and Schonbaum (Eds), Platelet, Drugs and Thrombosis (Karger, Basel, 1975).

6. Boston Collaborative Drug Surveillance Group. Regular aspirin intake and acute myocardial infarction. Brit. Med. J., 1, 440, 1974.

7. Brust, J.C.M. Transient ischemic attacks: Natural history and anticoagulation. Neurology, 24, 701, 1977.

8. Cobb, S., Anderson, F., Bauer, W. Length of life and cause of death in rheumatoid arthritis. New Engl. J. Med., 249, 553, 1953.

9. Coronary Drug Project Research Group: Clofibrate and niacin in coronary heart disease. JAMA, 231, 360, 1975.

10. Dale, J. Prevention of arterial thromboembolism with acetylsalicylic acid in patients with prosthetic heart valves. Thrombosis and Hemostasis, 38, 66, 1977.

11. Dyken, M.L., Kolar, O.J., Jones, F.M. Differences in the occurrence of carotid transient ischemic attacks associated with antiplatelet therapy. Stroke, 4, 732, 1973.

12. Ebert, R.V. The potential of anticoagulant treatment in acute myocardial infarction. Circulation Suppl., 40, 271, 1969.

13. Elwood, P.C., Cochrane, A.L., Burr, M.L., Sweetman, P.M., Williams, G., Welsby, E., Hughes, S.J., Renton, R. A randomized controlled trial of acetyl salicylic acid in the secondary prevention of mortality from myocardial infarction. Brit. Med. J., 1, 436, 1974.

14. Erhardt, L.R., Lundman, T., Mellstedt, H. Incorporation of ^{125}I-fibrinogen into coronary arterial thrombi in acute myocardial infarction. Lancet, 1, 387, 1973.

15. Evans, G. Effect of drugs that suppress platelet surface interaction on incidence of amaurosis fugax and transient inschemic attacks. Surgical Forum, 23, 239, 1972.

16. Feinstein, A.R. Clinical biostatistics. The clofibrate trials: another dispute about contratrophic therapy. Clin. Pharmacol. Ther., 13, 952, 1972.

17. Fields, W.G., Lemak, N.A., Frankowski, R.F., Hardy, R.J. Controlled trials of Aspirin in Cerebral Ischemia. Stroke, 8, 299, 1977.

18. Freed, M.D., Rosenthal, A., Fyler, D. Am. Heart J., 87, 283, 1974.

19. Friedli, B., Aerichide, N., Grondin, P., Campean, L. Thromboembolic complications of heart valve prosthesis. Am. Heart J., 81, 702, 1971.

20. Gadboys, H.L., Litwak, R.S., Niemetz, J., Wisch, N. Role of anticoagulants in preventing embolization from

prosthetic heart valves. JAMA, 202, 282, 1967.

21. Gent, A.E., Brook, C.G.D., Foley, T.H., Miller, T.N.
    Dipyridamole: a controlled trial of its effect in
    acute myocardial infarction. Brit. Med. J., 4, 366,
    1968.

22. Genton, E., Gent, M., Hirsh, J., Harker, L.A. Platelet
    inhibiting drugs in the prevention of clinical throm-
    botic disease. N. Engl. J. Med., 293, 1174, 1236,
    1296, 1975.

23. Gifford, R.M., Feinstein, A.R. A critique of methodo-
    logy in studies of anticoagulant therapy for acute
    myocardial infarction. N. Engl. J. Med., 280, 351,
    1969.

24. Group of Physicians of Newcastle-upon-Tyne Region:
    Trials of clofibrate in the treatment of ischaemic
    heart disease. Brit. Med. J., 4, 767, 1971.

25. Harker, L.A., Slichter, S.J. Platelet and fibrinogen
    consumption in man. New Engl. J. Med., 287, 999, 1972.

26. Harrison, M.J.G., Meadows, J.C., Marshall, J., Ross
    Russel, R.W. Effects of aspirin in amaurosis fugax.
    Lancet, 2, 743, 1971.

27. Heady, J.A. Bulletin World Health Organization, 48,
    243, 1973.

28. Hilden, T., Iversen, K., Raaschon, F., Schwartz, M.
    Anticoagulants in acute myocardial infarction. Lancet,
    2, 327, 1961.

29. Hynes, K.M., Gau, G.T., Rutherford, B.C., Kazmier,
    F.J., Frye, R.L. Effect of aspirin on brachial artery
    occlusion following brachial arteriotomy for coronary
    arteriography. Circulation, 47, 554, 1973.

30. International Anticoagulant Review Group: Collaborative
    analysis of long-term anticoagulant administration

after acute myocardial infarction. Lancet, 1, 203, 1970.

31. Loeliger, E.A., Hensen, A., Kroes, F., Van Dijk, L.M., Fekkes, N., De Jonge, H., Hemker, N.C. A double-blind trial of long-term anticoagulant treatment after myocardial infarction. Acta Med. Scand., 182, 549, 1967.

32. Master, A.M., Lassen, R.P. Transmural myocardial infarction. J. Amer. Ass., 209, 672, 1969.

33. McEnany, M.C., de Sanctis, R.W., Hawthrone, R.W. (Abstract): Circulation, 53, suppl. 2, 124, 1976.

34. Meuwissen, O.J.A.T., Vervoorn, A.C., Cohen, O., Jordan, F.L.J., Nelemans, F.A. Double-blind trial of long-term anticoagulant treatment after myocardial infarction. Acta Med. Scand., 186, 361, 1969.

35. Mundall, J., Quintero, P., von Kaulla, K.N., Harman, R., Austin, J. Transient ,olecular blindness and increased platelet aggregability treated with aspirin: A case report. Neurology, 22, 280, 1972.

36. Nicolaides, A.N., Kakkar, V.V., Renney, J.T.G., Kidner, P.H., Hutchinson, D.C.S., Clarke, M.B. Myocardial infarction and deep vein thrombosis. Brit. Med. J., 1, 432, 1971.

37. Packham, M.A., Mustard, J.F. Clinical Pharmacology of Platelets. Blood, 50, 555, 1977.

38. Preston, F.E., Emmanuel, I.G., Winfield, D.A., Malia, R.G. Essential thrombocythaemia and peripheral gangrene. Brit. Med. J., 3, 548, 1974.

39. Research Committee of the Scottish Society of Physicians. Ischemic heart disease: a secondary prevention trial using clofibrate. Brit. Med. J., 4, 775, 1971.

40. Roberts, W.C., Buja, L.M. The frequency and significance of coronary arterial thrombi and other obser-

vations in fatal acute myocardial infarction. Am. J.
Med., 52, 425, 1972.

41. Sullivan, J.M., Harken, D.E., Gorlin, R. Pharmacologic
control of thromboembolic complications of cardiac
valve replacement. New Engl. J. Med., 279, 579, 1968.

42. Tillgren, C., Stenson, S., Lund, F. Obliterative arterial disease of the lower limbs studied by means of
repeated femoral arteriography. Acta Radiol. (Stockholm), 1, 1161, 1963.

43. Verstraete, M. Are agents affecting platelet functions
clinically useful. Am. J. Med., 61, 897, 1976.

44. Veterans Administration Cooperative Clinical Trial:
Anticoagulants in Acute Myocardial Infarction. JAMA,
225, 724, 1973.

45. Vreeken, J., Van Aken, W.G. Spontaneous aggregation of
blood platelets as a cause of idiopathic thrombosis
and recurrent painful toes and fingers. Lancet, 2,
1394, 1971.

46. Weily, H.S., Steele, P.P., Davies, H., Pappas, G.,
Genton, E. Platelet survival in patients with substi-
tute heart valves. New Engl. J. Med., 290, 534, 1974.

47. Weiss, H.J. Antiplatelet drug. Am. Heart J., 92, 86,
1976.

48. Weiss, H.J. Platelet physiology and abnormalities of
platelet function. New Engl. J. Med., 293, 531, 580,
1975.

49. Working Party on Anticoagulant Therapy in Coronary
Thrombosis: Assessment of short-term anticoagulant
administration after cardiac infarction. Brit. Med. J.,
1, 335, 1969.

50. Wright, I.S., McDevitt, E. Cerebrovascular disease.
Ann. Intern. Med., 41, 682, 1954.

51. Wright, I.S., Marple, C., Beck, D. Report of the
    committee for the evaluation of anticoagulants in the
    treatment of coronary thrombosis with myocardial in-
    farction. Am. Heart J., _36_, 801, 1948.

Addendum

    After this review was completed the results of the
Canadian Cooperative Study Group (New Engl.J.Med. 299, 53,
1978) on a randomized trial of aspirin and sulphinpyrazone
in 585 patients with threatened stroke were published.
Aspirin reduced the risk of continuing ischemic attacks,
stroke and death by 19 percent. No such benefit was observed
for sulphinpyrazone. In addition no overall synergism or
antagonism between aspirin and sulphinpyrazone was shown.
It is of interest to note that the beneficial effect of
aspirin on the risk reduction for stroke and death was 48
percent in men whereas no significant trend was demonstrated
for women with threatened stroke. The reason for this sex
difference is unclear.

CLOSING REMARKS
Reitsma, W.D.

During this postgraduate course the various aspects
that, as far as we know at this time, are of importance in
the development of atherosclerosis, have been reviewed.
They include smoking, the use of oral contraceptives and
probably oral antidiabetic agents, the existence of hypertension, diabetes mellitus, some other endocrine diseases
like myxedema and Cushing's disease, hyperlipoproteinemia
and possibly abnormal platelet function. By the changing
habits in the way of living these risk factors became also
very relevant in the development of atherosclerotic diseases at Curaçao and the whole surrounding area.

All the different factors and diseases related to
atherosclerosis have been discussed with an emphasis on
the pathophysiological mechanisms, that may stimulate the
development of atherosclerosis. In the case of hypertension
the sequence of alterations that result in essential hypertension, has been explained. The relation between carbohydrate intolerance and triglyceride metabolism in diabetes mellitus and the effect of normalization of blood
glucose on microangiopathy have already been the subject
of many symposia. Recent developments are the recognition
of the L.D.L.-receptor, its impact on intracellular cholesterol metabolism and its significance in familial hyper-

cholesterolemia. Also a new area of interest is the role
of platelet adherence to places of endothelial damage resulting in release of platelet growth factor and stimulation of smooth muscle cell proliferation.

All the single aspects of the research in the field
of atherosclerosis are like pieces of a difficult puzzle.
Nowadays it seems that we are starting to understand some
interrelationships and that we are able to fit some pieces
of the puzzle together. The place of drugs that intervene
with platelet function still needs to be established. Future therapeutic approach may be directed upon the possibilities of stimulation of cholesterylester hydrolase enzymes, inhibition of the synthesis of cholesterylesters
and intervention with the reactions of the arterial wall.
However, in this moment these suggestions are still dreams
of the future.

As the main goal of this course is postgraduate teach-
ing, we paid much attention to the clinical manifestations of atherosclerosis, its diagnostic possibilities and
the established therapeutical approach. Despite the rapid
progress in fundamental research, in sophisticated diagnostic procedures and in the treatment of the acute complications of myocardial infarction, the treatment and especially the prevention of atherosclerotic manifestations remains disappointing. It has been stressed during this course that the adherence to a prescribed drug regime remains
a difficult problem especially during long term treatment
of patients with minor clinical symptoms. This makes it
understandable why it is nearly impossible to persuade
healthy people to abandon some agreable aspects of life,

238

which are known as risk factor in the development of atherosclerosis. Nevertheless this is the best, the most logic
and least expensive way to slow down the process of atherosclerosis.